国際学会 English
口頭発表
研究発表のための英語プレゼンテーション

C.S.Langham（日本大学特任教授）著

Presentation update:

A guide to starting, changing formal English to informal English, improving slides, enhancing the clarity of the main body, finishing, creating a clear summary slide, and writing an audience-friendly script

医歯薬出版株式会社

This book is originally published in Japanese
under the title of :

KOKUSAI GAKKAI INGURISSHU KOTO HAPPYO
(Presentation Update)

C. S. Langham
  Professor at Nihon University School of Dentistry

© 2019 1st ed.

ISHIYAKU PUBLISHERS, INC.
  7-10, Honkomagome 1 chome, Bunkyo-ku,
  Tokyo 113-8612, Japan

Introduction

This book is for people who need to give oral presentations in English. It is written in English and has section titles and short summaries of the main points in Japanese. The contents can be used in most fields and situations. My intention has been to provide a highly practical guide with numerous examples. I have attempted to make the material as accessible as possible and have avoided long explanations.

This book covers the following topics: **starting a presentation, using informal English that is suitable for an oral presentation, simple ways of improving slides, improving clarity in the main body of the presentation, finishing your presentation,** and **creating clear summary slides and an audience-friendly script.**

I would stress that readers should not feel they have to use all of the advice and examples in this book. It is necessary to be selective and choose the material that fits your presentation. I hope that readers of this book will find the contents useful and be able to improve their presentations.

Acknowledgments

Thanks are due to my colleagues at the Journal of Oral Science, particularly Professor N. Koshikawa, Editor in Chief, who has shown an interest in my work. I am indebted to Dr. Noriko Yamaguchi of the Institute of Agro-environmental Sciences for allowing access to presentation material. I also wish to acknowledge my colleague and friend, Brian Purdue of Tsukuba University, who has been a constant source of inspiration. Additionally, I have received support and advice from Michio Tajima and Minoru Hirata at Nihon University School of Dentistry. Finally, I wish to acknowledge the participants on presentation skills programs at the National Institute of Advanced Industrial Science and Technology and Tsukuba Center for Institutes.

Clive Langham
Nihon University
School of Dentistry
Ochanomizu, Tokyo
December 1st, 2019

Contents

Part 1   Starting
発表の始め方

1

自己紹介の仕方, 発表テーマや概略の説明の仕方など, 発表を始める際によく使われる表現と例文を紹介します.

1   Thank the Chairperson   ······2
座長へのお礼の挨拶

2   State your name and affiliation   ······3
名前と所属を述べる

3   Handling the title of your presentation   ······6
タイトルを紹介する

4   Using an overview slide to introduce the structure and contents of your presentation   ······10
目次スライドを活用して発表の構成を示す

5   How to introduce an overview slide using the words first, next, then, after that, in part 3, in the next part / section, finally, lastly   ······17
目次スライドの紹介に用いる接続表現

6   How to introduce an overview slide   ······20
目次スライドを紹介する

7   How to show the title, your name, affiliation, and an overview of the contents on one slide   ······27
タイトル, 名前・所属, 目次を1枚のスライドで紹介する

8   Starting without an overview slide: a short overview that provides a snapshot of the topic   ······31
目次スライドを使わずに発表を始める

9   Introduce the background   ······42
研究背景を紹介する

10   How to start a presentation as an invited speaker   ······49
招待講演の始め方

11   Useful sentences for: Thanking the audience for coming, Making informal opening comments, Giving a series of talks, Comments when you present after a well-known presenter, Dealing with technical problems   ······53
便利な表現集

V

Part 2　Using informal, spoken English to simplify and shorten the main body　59
話し言葉の英語を活用して簡潔な原稿を作成する方法

論文調の書き言葉の英語を，口頭発表に適した話し言葉の英語に変換する方法を紹介します．

1 How to reduce the level of formality in your presentation　……60
書き言葉の英語を話し言葉の英語に変換する方法

Part 3　Simple ways to improve your slides　83
スライド改善のポイント

スライド作成の際に注意したい，文法や英語表現に関する11のポイントを紹介します．

1 Number your slides　……84
スライドに番号をつけよう

2 A space is needed between a number and a word　……85
数字・記号と単語の間にはスペースが必要

3 Use the slide title box to show the section　……86
スライドの最上部のスペースを上手に活用しよう

4 Use of the definite article **the** in slide titles　……87
スライドタイトル中の定冠詞 **the** の使い方に注意しよう

5 Using contractions on slides: These samples **aren't** biodegradable　……88
スライドでは短縮形を使わないようにしよう

6 Slide title: Singular or plural? 's' or no 's'?　……89
スライドタイトルは単数形？ それとも複数形？

7 The word **of** can be a problem　……90
前置詞 **of** の使い方に注意しよう

8 Avoid using the words **my** or **our** in slides　……92
スライドでは **my** や **our** を用いるのはやめよう

9 Exclamation marks are not used in academic presentations or written papers
エクスクラメーションマークは学会発表では使用しない　……93

10 Problems with question marks: Is this a statement or a question?　……94
クエスチョンマークの誤用に注意しよう

11 Summary sentences at the bottom of slides: How to reduce the number of words
スライド下部に簡単なまとめを入れよう　……96

vi　Contents

Part 4 | # How to improve the clarity of the main body 101
本論を分かりやすく伝える方法

論理展開を示す表現，スライド内の情報を説明する表現など，本論（main body）の説明に必要な表現と例文を紹介します．

1 Starting a new topic, section 102
新しい話題／セクションを始める

2 Explaining what is on a slide 106
スライド内の情報を説明する

3 How to use the word mean 115
動詞 mean の正しい使い方

4 Useful expressions for explaining technical terms: by X, I mean, what do I mean by X?, in other words, X is defined as, I'm going to refer to X as Y 118
専門用語を説明する

5 Simplifying and rephrasing the information you present 123
情報を単純化して伝える／平易な表現に言い換える

6 Giving an estimate using the words about, approximately, in the region of, typical, typically, basically 127
詳細には触れず，おおまかな数値／一般論を述べる

7 Skipping information and focusing on the main points 131
要点の説明に絞り，一部の説明を省略する

8 How to help the audience follow your presentation by using forward movement, backward movement, and reminders 136
次に話す内容を予告する／前に話した内容を振り返る

9 Focusing on information on the slide 143
スライドのどこに注目してほしいかを示す

10 Focusing on results 151
結果と考察を説明する

11 Introducing references 164
参考文献を示す／結果を先行研究と比較する

12 Summarizing at 3 levels: one slide, several slides, a section 169
発表の途中にまとめを挟む：スライド1枚のまとめ，スライド数枚分のまとめ，セクションのまとめ

13 From data to explanation and implications 172
結果を考察する：結果が何を意味しているか／どのような意義をもつか

14 Introducing and explaining a video clip 174
動画を再生する

15 Time management, correcting yourself, correcting an error on a slide 178
発表時間の管理／発言内容とスライド内容の訂正

16 How to use the expressions stand for and is short for to introduce an acronym
アクロニム（頭字語）を説明する 180

17 Giving examples using **such as**, **for example**, **for instance** 181
具体例を挙げて説明する

18 Explaining a process using the words **first**, **next**, **after that**, **then** 183
手順を説明する

Part 5 Finishing your presentation
発表の終わり方 185

発表の終わり方の流れを16のステップに分けて紹介します．

1 Starting the summary: Steps 1-5 188
まとめを始める：ステップ1〜5

2 Introduce the findings, implications, and future work: Steps 6-11 194
研究結果のポイントや聴衆へのメッセージを述べる：ステップ6〜11

3 Finishing the presentation: Steps 12-16 204
発表を終える：ステップ12〜16

Part 6 How to create a clear summary slide and an audience-friendly script
分かりやすいまとめスライドの作り方，説明の仕方 209

簡潔で見やすいまとめスライド(summary slide)を作成する方法と，まとめスライドを説明する際の原稿作成のポイントを解説します．

1 Summary slide example 1 210
まとめスライドの改善例（1）

2 Summary slide example 2 220
まとめスライドの改善例（2）

Columns

#01 The word **my** is frequently misused 16
My の誤用に注意しよう

#02 I'll just **run through** / **go over** the main points 57
Run through, **go over** を上手に使おう

#03 A summary-box and mini-summary can help the audience follow your presentation 98
Summary-box と **mini-summary** を活用しよう

#04 Is it okay to read from the text on your computer? 184
口頭発表で原稿を読み上げるのは問題か？

viii Contents

Part 1
Starting
発表の始め方

Starting is one of the most important parts of your presentation. You have about a minute to introduce yourself, give the title of your presentation, and explain the material you will cover. In this section, I show how to start.

　口頭発表の始めには，座長へのお礼と自分の所属・名前を述べた後，発表のテーマや概略を簡潔に紹介します．その際，発表の構成を1枚にまとめた「目次スライド」を提示することもあります．この章では，発表を始める際によく使われる表現と例文を紹介します．

Thank the Chairperson
座長へのお礼の挨拶

Here are some examples of how to thank the Chairperson.

ご紹介ありがとうございます.

1. Thank you.
2. Thank you, Chair.
3. Thank you, Chairperson.
4. Thank you, Professor Williams.
5. Thank you for the introduction.
6. Thank you for your kind introduction.

一番短い1の例文が最もよい. 学会発表では, 短い文章が望ましい.

Example 1 is better because it is shorter and easier to say.

Common errors──よくある間違い

At a domestic conference I attended, several presenters started like this.

✗ Thank you *for the* Chairperson.

This sentence is incorrect. The expression, **thank you for**, is used like this.

○ Thank you **for the introduction**.
○ Thank you **for your kind introduction**.

In the question and answer session, **Thank you for**, is used like this.

○ **Thank you for** your question.
○ **Thank you for** the question.

Thank you for the chairperson という表現は誤り. Thank you for の後には, the introduction や your question などのように, 人ではなく行為が続く.

Part 1 ● Starting 発表の始め方

2 State your name and affiliation
名前と所属を述べる

Many presenters use difficult expressions and make basic grammatical mistakes when **stating their name and affiliation**. Here is a quick, easy to use example.

> 〜と申します． ○○大学の△△学部に所属しています．
>
> ▮ Thank you. <u>My name is</u> Ken Watanabe. <u>I'm with</u> London University. <u>I'm in</u> the Department of Informatics.

名前と所属を述べるのに，難しすぎる表現や，文法的に誤った表現を使っている人も多い．

The presenter introduces his/her affiliation using the simple expression, **I'm with** + affiliation.
It is also possible to say,

▮ <u>I work at</u> Osaka General Hospital.
▮ <u>I'm working at</u> Osaka General Hospital.
▮ <u>I'm at</u> Osaka General Hospital.

所属する大学や研究機関を述べるときは **I'm with** や **I work at** を用いる．

Please note that the word **department** is introduced with the preposition **in**.

▮ <u>I'm in</u> the Department of Informatics.
▮ <u>I'm in</u> the Department of Community Health.

学部名や部門名については **I'm in** で紹介する．

You can combine the following two sentences like this.

1 I'm with London University. **2** I'm in the Department of Informatics.

1+2 <u>I'm with</u> London University <u>in the</u> Department of Informatics.

I'm with（＋大学名）と **in**（＋学部名）を一文にまとめることもできる．

Using the words <u>with</u> and <u>in</u>, you can state your affiliation quickly and easily in a single sentence.

2 State your name and affiliation 名前と所属を述べる 3

Common errors——よくある間違い

✗ I am *staff* at Newcastle University.
✗ I am *a staff* at Newcastle University.
○ **I am a member of staff** at Newcastle University.

✗ I *work* Newcastle University.
○ **I work at** Newcastle University.

✗ I *work for* Newcastle University.
○ **I'm with** Newcastle University.

The verb **work for** is usually used with a company name, not a university or institute. Here is an example. **I work for Toyota**.

✗ I *belong to* Newcastle University.
○ **I'm with** Newcastle University.

✗ I'm *from* Newcastle University.
○ **I'm with** Newcastle University.

The pattern **I'm from** should not be used when stating your affiliation.

Please note that the following sentences using the word **from** are correct and can be used in general conversation.

○ **A speaker from London University** gave a very impressive presentation.
○ **There are a lot of people from Tokyo University** at this conference.

所属を説明する際，*I am（a）staff at* という表現は誤り．Staff を使う場合は **I am a member of staff at** とする．

Work for は通常企業名を紹介する際に用い，大学名・研究機関名には用いない．大学名を言いたいときは **work at** とする．

I'm from（＋大学名） は自分の所属の紹介としては誤り．ただし，他の研究者を **a speaker from（＋大学名）** と紹介することはできる．

4　Part 1 ●Starting　発表の始め方

Key points

1. After the Chairperson has introduced you, <u>Thank you</u> is the easiest way of starting.
2. *Thank you for the Chairperson* is incorrect.
3. Save time by stating your affiliation with the short, easy to say expression <u>I'm with + affiliation</u>.
4. If you want to include your department, division, or section, you can use the following sentence.
   - **I'm in + department, division, section.**
5. You can combine the two patterns <u>I'm with + affiliation</u> and <u>I'm in the department of</u> like this.
   - **I'm with London University <u>in</u> the Department of Informatics.**

・はじめに座長へのお礼を述べる．Thank you のような簡潔な表現が望ましい．

・続いて名前と所属を，I'm with（＋大学名，機関名），I'm in（＋学部名，部門名）などの表現で紹介する．

2 State your name and affiliation 名前と所属を述べる

3 Handling the title of your presentation
タイトルを紹介する

At domestic conferences in Japan, presenters read their presentation title in full. This wastes time because the title is in the conference handbook, has been announced by the Chairperson, and is also on the first slide. At international conferences, most presenters introduce the topic of their presentation by focusing on 2 or 3 keywords from the title, and do not read the title in full. Here is an example.

発表の正式なタイトルはプログラムやタイトルスライドに記載されているため，口頭で読み上げる必要はない．タイトルからキーワードをいくつか抜き出し，**I'm going to talk about**（＋キーワード）の形で示すとよい．

左の例のように，口頭で読み上げる内容は，スライドに表示される正式なタイトルよりも短くする．

Title
A clinicopathological study of salivary gland cancers
Script
Today, **I'm going to talk about** salivary gland cancers.

The presenter focuses on 3 words from the title, **salivary gland cancers** and introduces the topic with **Today, I'm going to + talk about + topic**.

Here are some more examples of how to introduce the title of your presentation.

本日は〜についてお話しします．

- Today, I'm going to <u>talk about</u> + 2 or 3 words from the title or a short, simplified version of the title.
- Today, I will <u>focus on</u> + 2 or 3 words from the title.
- My presentation today <u>is on</u> + 2 or 3 words from the title.
- My presentation today <u>is about</u> + 2 or 3 words from the title.
- This presentation <u>is about</u> + 2 or 3 words from the title.

6　Part I ● Starting　発表の始め方

3.1 Sentence structures for introducing titles
発表テーマ紹介のための構文

The following examples show common sentence structures for introducing the topic of your presentation.

- **I'm going to** talk about（topic）
- **I want to** talk about（topic）
- **I would（I'd）** like to talk about（topic）
- **I will（I'll）** talk about（topic）
- **I will（I'll）** be talking about（topic）
- **My presentation（today）is on**（topic）
- **This presentation is on**（topic）
- **My presentation（today）is about**（topic）

The most frequently used structure is **I'm going to talk about** + topic.

> **Note** In the above sentences, it is possible to say **I'm going to** or **I am going to**. Most native speakers will choose **I'm**, but it is also correct to say **I am**. If you are worried about pronunciation and want to avoid **I'm** or **I'd**, it is possible to introduce the presentation topic with these sentences.
>
> - **My/this presentation** is on + topic.
> - **My/this presentation** is about + topic.
> - **Today, I want to talk about** + topic.

発表テーマの紹介は，**I'm going to talk about**（＋キーワード）などの形が一般的である．

I'm, I'd の短縮形の発音に自信がない場合は，省略せずに I am, I would としたり，代わりに左記のような表現を用いるとよい．

3.2 Commonly used verbs for introducing a topic
発表テーマ紹介に用いる動詞

The three most common verbs for introducing a topic are: **talk about**, **focus on**, **look at**.

talk about 以外にも，focus on や look at を使うのもよい．

- I'm going to <u>talk about</u> recent developments in orthodontic techniques.
- I'm going to <u>focus on</u> the use of CAD/CAM in implant technology.
- I'm going to <u>look at</u> the use of CAD/CAM in implant technology.

The most frequent verb for introducing a topic is **talk about**. **Focus on** is also widely used. The verb **look at** is widely used by native speakers. **Look at** is an informal verb.

3.3 How to thank the Chairperson, state your name, affiliation, and topic
座長へのお礼→名前・所属→発表テーマ紹介の例

Here are two examples that include the following 3 functions.

1. Thanking the chairperson
2. Giving your name, affiliation and department
3. Stating the topic of the presentation

これまで説明した「座長へのお礼の挨拶」「自分の名前と所属の紹介」「タイトルの紹介」をつなげると、下記のようになる。

Script(座長へのお礼 → 名前・所属 → 発表テーマ紹介の例)

Example 1
Thank you for the introduction. I'm Neil Smith. I'm with Rutgers University in the Department of Orofacial Pain. Today, I'm going to focus on the trigeminal nerve.

Example 2
Thank you. My name's Chris Jones. I work at the University of Health Sciences in Brisbane. Today, I'll be talking about issues affecting public health.

Common errors——よくある間違い

✕ *Today's my topics* is about development of biodegradable polymers.

There are two errors in this sentence. First, *today's* does not need an apostrophe, and *s* should be deleted. Second, *topics* does not need an *s* as you will only be talking about one main theme or topic. It is better to change *topic* to *presentation* or *talk*. This sentence can be rewritten as follows.

○ <u>Today, my presentation is on/about</u> development of biodegradable polymers.
○ <u>My presentation today is on/about</u> development of biodegradable polymers.
○ <u>Today, my talk is on/about</u> development of biodegradable polymers.
○ <u>Today, I'm going to talk about / focus on</u> development of biodegradable polymers.

タイトルやトピックを紹介する際，*Today's my topics is* という表現は誤りである。Today のアポストロフィーは不要．また発表のメインテーマ1つについて述べる際は topic は単数形で用いる．この場合，topic よりも presentation や talk のほうが適している．

Key points

1. At international conferences, presenters do not read the presentation title in full.
2. Introduce your topic by focusing on <u>2 or 3 keywords</u> that are in the title.
3. The most common sentence for introducing the presentation topic is:
   - **Today, I'm going to talk about + topic.**
4. The most common pattern is: <u>I'm going to</u>
5. The most common verb is <u>talk about</u>. Other frequently used verbs are <u>focus on</u> and <u>look at</u>.

タイトル全体の読み上げは必要ない．タイトルからキーワードを 2，3 個抜き出して，I'm going to talk about（＋キーワード）などの形で紹介する．

3 Handling the title of your presentation　タイトルを紹介する

Using an overview slide to introduce the structure and contents of your presentation
目次スライドを活用して発表の構成を示す

The purpose of an overview slide is to **show the structure and contents** of your presentation. Some presenters return to this slide several times during the presentation. Common titles for the overview slide are as follows: **contents, overview, outline**. Please note that the word **contents** is plural and that **content** without **s** is incorrect as the title of an overview slide. Also, **overview**, **outline** and **background** should always be singular. You cannot say *overviews*, *outlines* or *backgrounds*. **Overview** and **outline** are always one word.

目次スライド（overview slide）の目的は，発表全体の構成を示すことである．発表の最初に示すだけではなく，発表の途中でも映すことで，全体の構成を振り返ることができるようにする発表者もいる．

目次スライドのスライドタイトルは，overview の他に，contents や outline としてもよい．contents は必ず複数形，overview や outline, background は必ず単数形とすることに注意する．

4.1 How to introduce an overview slide
目次スライドの紹介の仕方

Example 1: Here is an overview slide. The script is shown below.

Slide(目次スライドの例)

Community health interventions for pre-diabetics

Overview

1. Introduction to community health interventions
   ・How they work
   ・Typical users
2. Interventions for pre-diabetics
   ・Face-to-face
   ・Online
3. Data from a recent community health project
4. Summary and future directions

Part I ● Starting　発表の始め方

This is the supporting script to introduce the overview slide.

Script（前ページの目次スライドの紹介例）

1. State your name, affiliation, and title of the presentation 名前, 所属, タイトル

① Thank you. I'm Ken Wilson. I'm with King's College London in the Department of Community Health. ② I'm going to talk about community health interventions, particularly for people who are pre-diabetic.

2. Introduce the overview slide　目次スライドの紹介

③ This is an outline. ④ I'll start with an introduction to community health interventions, focusing on how they work and typical users. ⑤ I'll move on to interventions for pre-diabetics. These are face-to face and also online. ⑥ Then I'll show you some data from a recent community health project. ⑦ I'll finish with a summary and mention future directions.

> **Note** If you want to **add another topic to the overview slide**, use this sentence. **I'll also look at / focus on + topic.** This is the simplest way of adding a topic. You can repeat the same sentence several times.

Key sentences

1. Thank the Chairperson. State your name and affiliation 座長へのお礼, 名前・所属の紹介

ご紹介ありがとうございます．～大学の～と申します．

■ Thank you. I'm Ken Wilson. **I'm with** King's College, London in the Department of Community Health.

Examples

■ Thank you. I'm Ken Wilson. **I work at** Kings College, London in the Department of Community Health.

■ Thank you. I'm Ken Wilson. **I'm at** Kings College, London in the Department of Community Health.

目次スライドの紹介の前に，座長へのお礼や自己紹介を行う（pp. 2〜5 参照）.

4 Using an overview slide to introduce the structure and contents of your presentation
目次スライドを活用して発表の構成を示す

2. State the topic　発表テーマの紹介

本日は〜について発表いたします.

■ I'm going to <u>talk about</u> community health interventions, particularly for people who are pre-diabetic.

> Examples

■ I'm going to <u>focus on</u> community health interventions.

■ I'm going to <u>look at</u> community health interventions.

タイトル，発表テーマの紹介については pp. 6〜9 も参照.

3. Introduce the overview slide　目次スライドの提示

（目次スライドを提示して）こちらが本日お話しする内容です.

■ <u>This is an outline</u>.

> Examples

■ <u>This is an overview</u>.

■ <u>Here are</u> the contents.

■ <u>These are</u> the contents.

■ <u>This slide shows</u> the contents.

■ <u>These are the points, topics, contents</u> that <u>I am going to cover today</u>.

■ Today, <u>I'll be covering</u> these points/topics.

■ Today, <u>I'll be covering</u> the following points/topics/contents.

■ Today, <u>I'm going to cover these topics</u>.

■ <u>These are the topics I'm going to be covering</u>.

目次スライドの紹介を始める合図として，左記のような表現を用いる.

<u>Cover</u> is a useful verb to introduce information in an overview slide. For example, **This is an overview. These are the points I am going to cover today.** The word <u>cover</u> means <u>talk about</u>, <u>focus on</u>, <u>look at</u>.

目次スライドを示しながら「本日はこれらの内容についてお話しします」と言いたいときは，動詞 cover を用いると便利である.

12　**Part 1** ● Starting　発表の始め方

Note After using any of the sentences in section **3. Introduce the overview slide**, you can then read the information in the overview directly from the powerpoint slide. Please remember to use the pointer as you introduce the points on the slide. Using just one example sentence from section 3. will improve the start of your presentation. It will also help you to start your presentation with confidence.

目次スライドを提示した後は，レーザーポインターで指しながら，項目を1つ1つ読み上げていけばよい.

4. Introduce part 1 of the overview slide
目次スライドの紹介（1）

はじめに，〜についてご紹介します.

▌ **I'll start with** an introduction to community health interventions, <u>focusing on</u> how they work and typical users.

「最初に〜について紹介します」と言いたいときは，**I'll start with an introduction to** などの表現を用いる. **Introduction** の後ろは of ではなく **to** であることに注意する.

Examples

▌ **I'll begin with** an introduction to community health interventions, <u>looking at</u> how they work and typical users.

▌ **I'll start by looking at** community health interventions, <u>focusing on</u> how they work and typical users.

▌ **First, I'll introduce** community health interventions, <u>looking at</u> how they work and typical users.

▌ **First, I'll look at** community health interventions, <u>focusing on</u> how they work and typical users.

▌ **First, I'll look at** community health interventions, <u>concentrating on</u> how they work and typical users.

Note I'll begin with an <u>introduction to</u> NOT an *introduction of*. The correct preposition to use with **introduction** is **to**. Here is an example.

▌ I'll start with <u>an introduction to</u> community health interventions.

④ **Using an overview slide to introduce the structure and contents of your presentation**
目次スライドを活用して発表の構成を示す

5. Introduce part 2 of the overview slide
目次スライドの紹介（2）

続いて，〜についてお話しします.

■ **I'll move on to** interventions for pre-diabetics. These are face-to face and also online.

> **Examples**

■ **I'll go on to** interventions for pre-diabetics.

■ **Next, I'll look at / focus on / describe / explain** interventions for pre-diabetics.

次のトピックの紹介に移る際は move on to や go on to を用いるとよい.

The useful 3-word verbs **move on to** and **go on to** can be used to introduce the next section / theme / topic / point. The informal 2-word verbs **look at** and **focus on** are also useful for introducing a new topic. Even if you have used **look at** and **focus on** to introduce the title of the presentation, the same verbs can be used here again. Repetition of verbs, such as **look at** and **focus on**, is not an issue.

トピックを紹介する際は look at や focus on も便利である. 口頭発表では，これらの動詞を繰り返し用いても問題ない（例：前の文で look at を用いた場合も，次の文でも look at を使用できる）.

6. Introduce part 3 of the overview slide
目次スライドの紹介（3）

さらに，〜についてもお話しします.

■ **Then I'll show you** some data from a recent community health project.

> **Examples**

■ **Then I'll introduce** some data from a recent community health project.

■ **Then I'll focus on** some data from a recent community health project.

■ **After that I'll focus on** some data from a recent community health project.

その次のトピックに移る際は，Then や After that を使用する.

7. Move on to the last part of the overview slide: Summary and future directions　目次スライドの最後：まとめと今後の展望

最後に，発表のまとめと今後の研究課題について述べます.

■ **I'll finish with** a summary and **mention future directions**.

発表の最後に，まとめと今後の展望を述べることを示す.

`Examples`

■ **I'll summarize** the main points and **touch on** future **studies / work / research**.

The expressions **future directions**, **future plans** and **future studies** are plural. But **future work** and **future research** are singular and should not be in used in the plural form. You cannot say *future works* or *future researches*. The expressions **future studies**, **future plans** and **future projects** are always plural in this context.

「今後の展望」「今後の研究課題」と言いたいとき，future studies, future plans, future projects は必ず複数形で，future work, future research は必ず単数形で用いることに注意する（p. 203 も参照）.

`Common errors──よくある間違い`

✕ This is *my* outline.
◯ This is an outline.

My という単語の使い方には注意が必要である. 詳しくは次ページのコラムを参照.

You should avoid using *my*. See page 16: Column, The word **my** is frequently misused.

✕ This is *today's* topics.
◯ This slide shows the contents of my presentation.

✕ This is *today's* contents.
◯ Here are the contents.

「本日の発表」と言いたいとき，*today's* という言い方は誤り. また topic よりも presentation や talk のほうがよい. p. 9 の Common errors も参照.

Also avoid using the word *today's*, as it is unnecessary. The words **presentation** and **talk** are more frequently used than **topic**. It is better to avoid the word **topic**.

④ Using an overview slide to introduce the structure and contents of your presentation
目次スライドを活用して発表の構成を示す

Column #01

The word my is frequently misused
My の誤用に注意しよう

Here are some common errors. In the following sentences, the use of the word <u>my</u> is unnatural and too informal.

✗ *This is my outline.*	◯ This is an outline.
✗ *This is my background.*	◯ This is some background.
✗ *Here are my contents.*	◯ These are the contents.
	◯ Here are the contents.
✗ *Here are my results.*	◯ Here are the results.
	◯ These are the results.
✗ *This is my summary.*	◯ This is a summary.
✗ *This is my conclusion.*	◯ This is the conclusion.
✗ *This is my apparatus.*	◯ This is the apparatus we used.
✗ *This is my hospital.*	◯ This is where I work.
✗ *This is my device.*	◯ This is the device we used.

However, please note the correct use of my in the following sentences.

◯ <u>My presentation today is about</u> + 2 or 3 words from the title.
◯ <u>My presentation is in 5 parts</u>.
◯ <u>This is my last slide</u>.

My はくだけた表現なので，学会発表の場で用いるには注意を要する．ただし，my presentation とするのは問題ない．

Part I ● Starting　発表の始め方

How to introduce an overview slide using the words first, next, then, after that, in part 3, in the next part / section, finally, lastly
目次スライドの紹介に用いる接続表現

5.1 How to emphasize the structure of the presentation
接続表現を活用して発表の構成を示す

When introducing an overview slide, some presenters emphasize the structure of the presentation using these words: **first**, **next**, **then**, **after that**, **in part 3**, **in the next part / section**, **finally**, **lastly**. Here is an example.

> 目次スライドを紹介する際，左記のような順序を表す接続表現を活用することで，発表全体の構成を強調することができる．

Script (接続表現を用いて発表の構成を明確にした原稿の例)

Today, I want to <u>focus on</u> a new concept of treating Parkinson's disease. My presentation is <u>in 5 main parts</u>. <u>First</u>, I'll <u>go over</u> the main causes of the disease and treatments of the disease. <u>Next</u>, I'll <u>explain</u> the concept of atypical anti-Parkinson compounds. <u>In part three</u>, I'll <u>discuss</u> the effects of a prototype. <u>After that</u>, I'll <u>consider</u> animal models, namely monkeys. <u>Finally</u>, I'll <u>focus on</u> sites of action in the brain.

In the above example, the presenter introduces the topic with **focus on**. **Today, I want to focus on（topic）**. The number of sections in the presentation is introduced like this. **My presentation is in 5 main parts** / **has 5 parts** / **is divided into 5 parts** / **consists of 5 parts**. The following verbs are used to introduce the sections. **go over** / **explain** / **discuss** / **consider** / **focus on**.

> 「本日の発表は○つのパートから構成されます」と言いたいときは，**My presentation is in 5 main parts** などと言うとよい．

5.2 How to introduce an overview slide using as few words as possible
より簡潔に目次スライドを紹介する

Some presenters <u>avoid the words used in 5.1 above</u> in order <u>to save time</u> and <u>simplify the explanation</u>. Instead they use the following verbs: **talk about, is, has, focus on, look at, mention**. Here is an example.

前ページの例よりも接続表現を減らし，より簡潔な表現とすることで，発表時間を有効に使うこともできる．

▍Script（語数を減らしてより簡潔な表現にした原稿の例）

<u>Today I am going to talk about</u> standards. <u>This is an outline.</u> <u>My presentation has 4 main parts.</u> <u>I'll focus on</u> problems with standard measurement systems and <u>look at</u> ways of adapting them. <u>I'll also look at</u> performance. Finally, <u>I'll look at</u> reliability tests and show you some of the data we got. <u>I'll also mention</u> future work.

> **Note** The presenter uses the two-word verb <u>look at</u> three times in this example. This saves time. This kind of repetition is not a problem in an oral presentation and is commonly used by native speakers. It is, of course, unacceptable in written academic English.

上記の原稿では **look at** という表現を何度も使っているが，口頭発表ではこのような繰り返しは問題にならない．もちろん，学術論文など書き言葉では許容されない．

Key points

1. An overview slide will help the audience to understand the structure and contents of the presentation.
2. The key functions to use when introducing an overview slide are as follows:
   - **This is an overview/outline.**
   - **Here are the contents.**
   - **These are the points I'll be covering today.**
3. Introduce the structure of the presentation
   - **My presentation is in 5 parts.**
4. Refer to each part of the contents slide
   - **I'll start with an introduction.**
   - **I'll look at（topic）.**
   - **I'll focus on（topic）.**
   - **I'll move on to（topic）.**
   - **I'll finish with a summary.**
5. Commonly used verbs for introducing the parts of an overview slide are as follows: start with, look at, focus on, move on to, finish with.
6. Some presenters use words such as first, next, then, after that, in part 3, in the next part / section, finally, lastly to introduce an overview slide. These help to indicate the structure of the presentation as clearly as possible.
7. Other presenters save time by using expressions such as talk about, is, has, focus on, look at and mention. Some native speakers use the word look at several times when introducing the slide. Repeating the same verb look at several times to introduce the material on the overview slide is not an issue.

・発表の最初に目次スライドを示すことで，聴衆は発表全体の構成をあらかじめ把握することができ，発表の内容を理解しやすくなる．

・目次スライド内の項目を１つ１つ紹介していく際は，look at や focus on などの句動詞を活用するとよい．Look at を繰り返し使っても問題ない．

・First，next など，順序を表す接続表現の活用も効果的である．

⑤ How to introduce an overview slide using the words first, next, then, after that, in part 3, in the next part / section, finally, lastly　目次スライドの紹介に用いる接続表現

6 How to introduce an overview slide
目次スライドを紹介する

Example 2: Here is an overview slide. The script is shown below.

Slide(目次スライドの例)

> **Role of iron plaque in controlling distribution and speciation of As and Cd in paddy soils**
>
> ## Overview
>
> 1. What is iron plaque?
> 2. Synchrotron micro-beam X-ray absorption
> 3. Distribution and speciation of As around iron plaque and iron mottle
> 4. Distribution and speciation of Cd around iron plaque
> 5. Conclusions and remaining questions

This is the supporting script to introduce the overview slide

Script(上記目次スライドの紹介例)

① Thank you for the introduction. My name is Jane Stevens. I'm with the University of Oxford. ② Today I will focus on the role of iron plaque. ③ As you can see, my presentation has 5 parts. ④ First, I'll ask the question: What is iron plaque? ⑤ Next, I'll move on to synchrotron micro-beam X-ray absorption. ⑥ Then, I will look at distribution and speciation of As around iron plaque and iron mottle. ⑦ I will also look at distribution and speciation of Cd around iron plaque. ⑧ I'll finish with some conclusions ⑨ and briefly mention remaining questions. ⑩ I'll start by focusing on iron plaque.

Part 1 ● Starting 発表の始め方

Key sentences

1. Thank the chairperson　座長へのお礼の挨拶

ご紹介ありがとうございます.

▌ **Thank you for the introduction**.

Examples

▌ **Thank you**.

▌ **Thank you, Chair**.

▌ **Thank you, Chairperson**.

▌ **Thank you, Professor Suzuki**.

▌ **Thank you for your kind introduction**.

2. Introduce the topic　発表テーマを紹介する

本日は〜について発表します.

▌ **Today, I will focus on** the role of iron plaque.

Examples

▌ **Today, I'll talk about** the role of iron plaque.

▌ **Today, I want to look at** the role of iron plaque.

▌ **In this presentation, I'll be talking about** the role of iron plaque.

▌ **In this presentation, I'll be focusing on** the role of iron plaque.

> **Note** The patterns **I'll talk about** and **I'll be talking about** have the same meaning. The frequency of **I'll talk about** is much higher than **I'll be talking about**.

6 How to introduce an overview slide　目次スライドを紹介する

3. Refer to the structure of the presentation
発表全体の構成を示す

本日の発表は○つのパートに分かれます．

▌ As you can see, my presentation has 5 parts.

Examples

▌ My presentation is in 5 parts.

▌ This presentation is divided into 5 parts.

▌ There are 5 parts in this presentation.

▌ This presentation has 5 parts.

▌ This presentation consists of 5 parts.

発表全体がいくつの
パートに分かれるかを
最初に示すことで，聴
衆が全体の構成を把握
しやすくなる．

4. Use a question to focus on the main topic
疑問形を使って発表テーマを紹介する

はじめに，皆さんに質問します．

▌ First, I'll ask the question: What is iron plaque?

Examples

▌ I'll start with the question: What is iron plaque?

▌ I'd like to begin by posing the question: What is iron plaque?

「～とは何でしょう
か？」のように疑問形
を用いて聴衆に問いか
けることで，発表のト
ピックを効果的に示す
ことができる．

Note The expression to pose a question is formal and means to ask a question.

5. Introduce the next section using the verb move on to
次の話題に移る（1）

次に，〜についてお話します．

▮ **Next, I'll move on to** synchrotron micro-beam X-ray absorption.

Examples

▮ **Next, I'll go on to** synchrotron micro-beam X-ray absorption.

▮ **Next, I'll look at** synchrotron micro-beam X-ray absorption.

▮ **Next, I'll consider** synchrotron micro-beam X-ray absorption.

▮ **Next, I'll introduce** synchrotron micro-beam X-ray absorption.

目次スライド内の次の項目の紹介へと移る際は，左記のように述べるとよい．

6. Introduce the next section with the verb look at
次の話題に移る（2）

それから，〜についてお話しします．

▮ **Then I will look at** distribution and speciation of As around iron plaque and iron mottle.

Examples

▮ **Then I will focus on** distribution and speciation of As around iron plaque and iron mottle.

▮ **After that I will talk about** distribution and speciation of As around iron plaque and iron mottle.

目次スライド内の各項目で発表するトピックを示す際には，**look at** や **focus on** などの句動詞を用いるとよい．

6 How to introduce an overview slide　目次スライドを紹介する

7. Introduce the next section with the verb look at
次の話題に移る（3）

〜についてもお話しします．

- **I will also look at** distribution and speciation of Cd around iron plaque.

Examples
- **I will also discuss**（topic）．
- **I will also consider**（topic）．

8. State how you will finish the presentation（1）
発表の終わり方を述べる（1）

最後にまとめと〜（9に続く）

- **I'll finish with some conclusions**（this sentence continues in 9. below）．

Examples
- **I'll conclude with** a summary...
- **Finally, I'll give** a brief summary...

発表の終わりに，まとめと今後の研究課題を紹介することを述べ，目次スライドの紹介を終わらせる．

9. State how you will finish the presentation（2）
発表の終わり方を述べる（2）

〜今後の研究課題についても述べたいと思います．

- ... and briefly **mention** remaining questions.

Examples
- ... and briefly **touch on** remaining questions.
- ... and **talk about** remaining issues.
- ... and **say something about** remaining issues.
- ... and **mention** future research.

今後の研究課題について言及することを示すときは，mention やtouch on を用いることが多い．

24　Part I ●Starting　発表の始め方

The following verbs are useful for introducing future research, future work, future plans, remaining issues, applications: **touch on**, **talk about**, **say something about**, **mention**.

10. Start part one of the presentation
    最初の話題に入ることを示す

> それでは，はじめに〜についてお話しします．
>
> ■ **I'll start by focusing** on iron plaque.
>
> ▸ Examples
> ■ **I'm going to start by talking about**（topic）．
> ■ **I'll start by looking at**（topic）．
> ■ **Let me start by describing**（topic）．

一通り発表の構成を示した後，発表の本題に入るときは左記のように言うとよい．

 The grammar pattern, **start / begin by + verb+ing** (start by talking about / looking at / focusing on), is useful for introducing topics.

Key points

1. Introduce the structure of the presentation by stating the number of points, themes, topics you will cover.
   - **My presentation is in 5 parts.**
   - **My presentation has 5 parts / is divided into 5 parts / consists of 5 parts.**
2. Use a question to introduce / focus on an important topic.
   - **First, I'll ask the question: What is iron plaque?**
3. Indicate a new section/part of the presentation with the following expressions:
   - **Next, I'll move on to**（topic）．
   - **Then I'll look at**（topic）．
   - **After that, I'll mention**（topic）．
   - **I'll also look at**（topic）．

6 How to introduce an overview slide 目次スライドを紹介する 25

4. State how you will finish the presentation. I'll finish with a summary and mention future work.
   Useful verbs for stating how you will finish the presentation:
   - **I'll finish with / conclude with a summary.**
   Useful verbs for referring to future work:
   - **I'll mention / touch on / say something about future work.**
5. Start part one of the presentation
   - **I'll start / begin by focusing on / talking about（topic）.**

・最初に発表全体がいくつのパートに分かれているかを示すとよい.

・発表テーマを紹介する際は，疑問形を使って聴衆に問いかけると効果的である.

・目次スライドの説明を終えた後は，I'll start by focusing on（topic）の形で本題に入る.

How to show the title, your name, affiliation, and an overview of the contents on one slide
タイトル，名前・所属，目次を１枚のスライドで紹介する

Some presenters **combine slides 1 and 2**. This means that the **first slide will contain the title, your name, affiliation, and an overview of the contents**. The advantage is that the audience can scan the information in slide 1 as you are talking.

タイトル・名前・目次のスライドと目次スライドを１枚にまとめる発表者もいる．こうすることによって，聴衆により効率的に情報を伝えることができる．

Here is an example.

Slide(タイトルスライドと目次スライドを1枚にまとめた例)

> **Characterization of radiocesium-bearing microparticles deposited and resuspended in Fukushima**
> Name and affiliation
>
> **Overview**
> 1. Forms of radiocesium released from FDNPs
> 2. What are radioactive particles?
> 3. Conclusions and future studies

Script(上記スライドを説明するための原稿例)

① <u>Thank you for the introduction</u>. (Name and affiliation) ② <u>Today I'll be talking about</u> radiocesium bearing micro-particles. ③ <u>Here are the contents</u>. ④ <u>I'll start by focusing on</u> forms of radiocesium released from FDNPs. ⑤ <u>Next, I'll ask</u> the question: What are radioactive particles? ⑥ <u>I'll finish with some conclusions</u> and <u>mention</u> future studies.

Key sentences

1. Thank the chairperson　座長へのお礼の挨拶

ご紹介ありがとうございます.

▌ **Thank you for the introduction**.

> Examples

▌ **Thank you**.
▌ **Thank you for your kind introduction**.

2. State the presentation topic　発表テーマを紹介する

本日は〜についてお話しします.

▌ **Today I'll be talking about** radiocesium bearing microparticles.

> Examples

▌ **I'm going to focus on** radiocesium bearing microparticles.
▌ **I'm going to be talking about** radiocesium bearing microparticles.
▌ **I want to look at** radiocesium bearing microparticles.
▌ **I'd like to talk about** radiocesium bearing microparticles.

3. Introduce the structure of the presentation
目次の紹介を始める

こちらが本日の発表の目次です.

▌ **Here are the contents**.

> Examples

▌ **Here / These are the contents**.
▌ **Here / These are the points / topics / things / areas I'm going to cover**.
▌ **These are the main points I'll cover today**.

発表テーマを紹介した後, 目次の紹介に移る合図として左記のような表現を用いるとよい.

28　Part Ⅰ ● Starting　発表の始め方

4. State the topic　目次スライド内の項目について説明する

はじめに〜についてお話しします.

- **I'll start by focusing on** forms of radiocesium released from FDNPs

  `Examples`
- **I'll begin by looking at** (topic).
- **First, I'll look at** (topic).
- **In part 1, I'll talk about** (topic).

目次スライドを単体で作成したとき同様，目次内の項目を順番に紹介していく.

5. Focus on a topic using a question
疑問形を使ってトピックを紹介する

次に，皆さんに質問をいたします.

- **Next, I'll ask the question**: What are radioactive particles?

  `Examples`
- **Next, I'll pose the question**: What are radioactive particles?

疑問形を用いて聴衆に問いかけることで，発表のトピックを聴衆に印象づけることができる.

6. State how you will finish the presentation
発表の終わり方を述べる

最後はまとめと今後の研究課題についてお話しします.

- **I'll finish with some conclusions and mention future studies.**

  `Examples`
- **I'll summarize the main points** and **touch on** future research.
- **I'll finish with a summary** and **talk briefly about** our ongoing work.

「(詳細には触れず) 簡単にお話しします」と言いたいときは，mention, touch on や talk briefly about と言うとよい.

---

7 **How to show the title, your name, affiliation, and an overview of the contents on one slide**
タイトル，名前・所属，目次を1枚のスライドで紹介する

29

Key points

1. It is possible to save time by combining slides 1 and 2.
2. This means that the first slide shows the <u>title</u>, your <u>name</u>, <u>affiliation</u> and an <u>overview of the contents</u>.
3. Remember that the audience will rapidly scan the information on slide 1 as you are speaking.

タイトル，名前・所属，目次を 1 枚のスライドにまとめることで，聴衆は発表者が話している間に一通りの情報を確認することができ，効率的な情報伝達が可能となる．

Starting without an overview slide: a short overview that provides a snapshot of the topic
目次スライドを使わずに発表を始める

Some experienced presenters tell me that they do not generally use an overview slide. Instead, they give <u>a short oral overview</u> that <u>provides a snapshot</u> of the topic and contents. Here are the reasons they give. **There is not enough time. Everyone knows the material. The audience can follow the contents of the presentation without an overview slide.** I have included the following example for presenters who do not want to use an overview slide.

目次スライドを作成せず，発表の概略を口頭で説明する発表者もいる。こうした方法は，目次スライドを紹介する時間がないとき，聴衆に十分な予備知識があるとき，目次スライドがなくても聴衆が発表の内容を理解可能なときに用いられる．

 8.1 A short overview that provides a snapshot of the topic without using a slide
目次スライドを使用しない発表の始め方（1）

> **Example 1**（目次スライドを使わずに発表の概略を説明する例 1）
>
> Thank you for the introduction. My name is Susan Hastings. <u>I'm with</u> London University in the Department of Community Medicine. ① <u>We have been working on</u> ways of helping people at high risk of diabetes. ② <u>Our main focus is</u> community projects where pre-diabetic people meet with health workers in the community. ③ <u>We are also interested in</u> creating online support material for such people. ④ <u>Currently, we are involved in</u> a project monitoring the health of 1,500 high-risk individuals enrolled in community support projects.
> ⑤ <u>Today I want to talk about</u> community health interventions. ⑥ <u>I'll start with some background.</u> ⑦ <u>Then I'll explain</u> how community projects were set up, and <u>talk about</u> the research we conducted.

Key sentences

1. Statement of general research area 研究領域を述べる

私達は○○（大まかな研究領域）の研究を行っています.

■ <u>We have been working on</u> ways of helping people at high risk of diabetes.

はじめに発表の背景として, 自分がどのような研究を行っているかを述べる.

Examples

■ We have been <u>doing research on</u> ways of helping people at high risk of diabetes.

■ We have been <u>focusing on</u> ways of helping people at high risk of diabetes.

■ We have been <u>looking at</u> ways of helping people at high risk of diabetes.

■ We have been <u>investigating</u> ways of helping people at high risk of diabetes.

研究領域を紹介するときは, We have been doing research on (+ topic) などと言う. *We are researching on* (+ *topic*) とするのは文法的に誤り. 現在進行形の We are doing research on (+ topic)や現在完了進行形の We have been doing research on (+ topic) とする.

Note In example 1, the following pattern is used: <u>We have been doing research on + topic</u>. Please note that the following expression is grammatically incorrect: *We are researching on* (*topic*). The correct pattern is: <u>do + research on + topic</u>. Here are 2 examples.

前置詞 on は, research on (+ topic) の他に, to research the effect of X on Y や This study was on (+ topic) などのパターンでも使用される.

■ <u>We have been doing research on</u> (topic).
■ <u>We are doing research on</u> (topic).

However, please note the following pattern. <u>We are researching the effect of sunlight on degradation rates</u>. The pattern is <u>to research the effect of X on Y</u>. The word <u>on</u> is also used in the following patterns. <u>This study was on</u> (topic). <u>This research was on</u> (topic). See p 74, Note We are studying *on*

32   Part 1 ● Starting　発表の始め方

2. Specific statement of topic　より具体的な研究テーマを紹介する

私達は特に，○○（具体的な研究テーマ）について研究しています．

- **Our main focus is** community projects where pre-diabetic people meet with health workers in the community.

  Examples
- **We are looking at** community projects where pre-diabetic people meet with health workers in the community.
- **We are working on** community projects where pre-diabetic people meet with health workers in the community.
- **We are focusing on** community projects where pre-diabetic people meet with health workers in the community.
- **We are particularly interested in** community projects where pre-diabetic people meet with health workers in the community.
- **The main focus of our work is** community projects where pre-diabetic people meet with health workers in the community.

大まかな研究領域を述べた後，より具体的な内容を説明する.

Note This is a short note on different patterns using the word **focus**. The example above uses the pattern, **The main focus of our work is** (+ topic).
The following patterns are also possible.

- **The main focus of our work is on** + topic.
- **Our main focus is on** + topic.
- **Our main focus is** + topic.
- **We are focusing on** + topic.

具体的な研究テーマを紹介するときは，**focus** を用いると便利である. **The main focus of our work is** (+ topic) の他にも，左記のような表現も用いられる.

⑧ Starting without an overview slide: a short overview that provides a snapshot of the topic
目次スライドを使わずに発表を始める

3. Further statement of topic　研究テーマをさらに紹介する

さらに，〜の研究も行っています.

- **We are also interested in** creating online support material for such people.

Examples

- **Additionally, we are developing** online support material for such people.
- **In addition, we are making** online support material for such people.

4. Statement of current research
現在の研究内容を具体的に述べる

現在，〜に関する研究計画を進めています.

- **(Currently), we are involved in** a project monitoring the health of 1,500 high-risk individuals enrolled in community support projects.

Examples

- **(Currently), we are developing** a project monitoring the health of 1,500 high-risk individuals enrolled in community support projects.
- **(At the moment), we are setting up** a project monitoring the health of 1,500 high-risk individuals enrolled in community support projects.
- **(Now,) we are creating** a project monitoring the health of 1,500 high-risk individuals enrolled in community support projects.
- **We are (now) creating** a project monitoring the health of 1,500 high-risk individuals enrolled in community support projects.

研究の現状（どのようなプロジェクトを進めているか）を紹介する.左記の例文のうち,（ ）内の文言は省略しても構わない.

Note In the above examples, the words in parentheses can be omitted.

5. Introduce the presentation topic　発表テーマを紹介する

本日は〜について発表いたします.

- **Today, I want to talk about** community health interventions.

  Examples
- **Today, I am going to focus on** community health interventions.
- **Today, I want to consider** community health interventions.
- **Today, I'll be looking at** community health interventions.
- **My presentation is about** community health interventions.
- **My presentation is on** community health interventions.

Note In the above preview, **the title / topic of the presentation is introduced at the end of the short overview and not at the beginning**. In function 5, the presenter introduces the topic of the presentation like this. **Today, I want to talk about** + topic. This means that in this type of overview, the position of the presentation title is flexible.

この例では，発表テーマ（タイトル）の紹介を研究内容の説明よりも後に行っている．このように，発表の概略を口頭で説明する場合には，発表テーマをいつ紹介するかを柔軟に変更することができる.

6. State that you will explain the background
背景を説明することを述べる

はじめに研究の背景についてお話しします.

- **I'll start with some background**.

  Examples
- **I'll give you** some background.
- **I'll explain** the background.
- **I'll mention** some background.
- **I'll start by explaining** some background.

発表テーマを紹介した後，発表の構成を順番に説明する.

8 Starting without an overview slide: a short overview that provides a snapshot of the topic
目次スライドを使わずに発表を始める

35

7. Introduce the next topic　次の話題に移る

> 続いて，〜について説明します．

- **Then I'll explain** how community projects were set up.

Examples
- After that **I'll tell you** how community projects were set up.
- Following that **I'll go over** how community projects were set up.

A short overview that provides a snapshot of the presentation without using a slide
目次スライドを使用しない発表の始め方 (2)

Example 2（目次スライドを使わずに発表の概略を説明する例 2）

Thank you. ① I'm Ken Williams. <u>I'm with</u> the University of Wales. <u>I'm in</u> the department of operative dentistry. ② <u>Today I'll be talking about</u> esthetic dentistry. ③ Over a number of years, <u>we have been focusing on</u> patient satisfaction levels. ④ We know that the number of people who want to improve the appearance of their teeth is increasing. ⑤ <u>But we don't know much about</u> levels of post-treatment patient satisfaction. ⑥ <u>We looked at</u> three commercial whitening products, ⑦ and <u>focused on</u> levels of patient satisfaction with those products. ⑧ <u>We wanted to see how</u> patients evaluated the products they used. ⑨ <u>I'd like to start with</u> some background.

Key sentences

1. Name and affiliation　名前と所属

〜大学の〜と申します.

- I'm Ken Williams. **I'm with** the University of Wales. **I'm in** the department of operative dentistry.

Examples

- **I'm at** the University of Wales. **I'm in** the department of operative dentistry.
- **I'm working at** the University of Wales. **I'm in** the department of operative dentistry.
- **I work at** the University of Wales. **I'm in** the department of operative dentistry.
- **I'm with** the University of Wales **in** the department of operative dentistry.

2. Introduce the topic　発表テーマの紹介

本日は〜について発表いたします.

- **Today I'll be talking about** esthetic dentistry.

Examples

- **I'm going to talk about** esthetic dentistry.
- **Today I'm going to focus on** esthetic dentistry.

この例では, Example 1とは異なり, 発表テーマを最初に紹介している.

> **Note** In this example, **the presenter introduces the title/topic in function 2**. In example 1, **the title was introduced in function 5 (see page 35),** which was later. This means that when giving a snapshot of the presentation, the position of the title/topic is flexible.

8 Starting without an overview slide: a short overview that provides a snapshot of the topic
目次スライドを使わずに発表を始める

3. State the main research area 研究領域を述べる

私達は〜について研究しています.

■ **Over a number of years, we have been focusing on** patient satisfaction levels.

Examples

■ **Our main subject of interest is** patient satisfaction levels.

■ **For several years, we have been looking at** patient satisfaction levels.

■ **For a number of years, we have been working on** patient satisfaction levels.

> **Note** It is possible to omit the following expressions: **over a number of years**, **for several years**, **for a number of years**. So, the shorter sentences without these expressions are as follows: **We have been focusing on / We have been looking at / We have been working on** + topic.

自分がどのような研究を行っているかを述べる. **Over a number of years** を省略し, より簡潔な文にすることもできる.

4. State the known information 既知の情報を説明する

先行研究によって, 〜であることが明らかになっています.

■ **We know that** the number of people who want to improve the appearance of their teeth is increasing.

Examples

■ **A lot of groups have reported that** the number of people who want to improve the appearance of their teeth is increasing.

■ **A lot of studies have reported that** the number of people who want to improve the appearance of their teeth is increasing.

■ **It is well known that** the number of people who want to improve the appearance of their teeth is increasing.

■ **It is well documented that** the number of people who want to improve the appearance of their teeth is increasing.

以下, 「○○についてはよく知られているが, △△についてはまだ分かっていないことが多い. そこで, △△について〜」という流れで, これから発表する研究の意義を紹介する.

はじめに, 先行研究によってどこまで明らかになっているのかを述べる.

5. State the unknown information（This is known as the research gap/niche） 研究ギャップ／ニッチを紹介する

しかし，〜についてはまだ分かっていません．

- **But we don't know much about** levels of post-treatment patient satisfaction.

Examples

- **However, we have no information on** levels of post-treatment patient satisfaction.
- **However, we have little information on** levels of post-treatment patient satisfaction.
- **However, there is little information on** levels of post-treatment patient satisfaction.
- **However, there is nothing on** levels of post-treatment patient satisfaction.
- **However, there are only a few studies on** levels of post-treatment patient satisfaction.
- **But, there is nothing in the literature on** levels of post-treatment patient satisfaction.
- **But, there is not much in the literature on** levels of post-treatment patient satisfaction.
- **However, there have been no reports in the literature on** levels of post-treatment patient satisfaction.
- **But, there have been few reports on** levels of post-treatment patient satisfaction.
- **However, few studies have focused on** levels of post-treatment patient satisfaction.

続いて「まだ分かっていないこと」を紹介する．

この「まだ分かっていないこと」は，research gap（研究ギャップ）や research niche（研究ニッチ）とよばれる．

However と But はどちらを使っても構わない．

In the literature の使い方，文献／先行研究に関するその他の表現については，p. 67 と p, 166 を参照．

 Note In all of the above examples, you can use either **however** or **but**.

 Note For more information on the phrase **in the literature**, please see pages 67 and 166.

8 Starting without an overview slide: a short overview that provides a snapshot of the topic
目次スライドを使わずに発表を始める

6. State research topic 1 研究内容を述べる (1)

~を調査しました.

- **We looked at** three commercial whitening products.

  Examples
- **We focused on** three commercial whitening products.
- **We investigated** three commercial whitening products.
- **We researched** three commercial whitening products.
- **We analyzed** three commercial whitening products.

6〜8 では，具体的にどのような研究を行ったのか，どのような目的で行ったのかを説明する.

7. State research topic 2 研究内容を述べる (2)

~についても調査しました.

- **We focused on** levels of patient satisfaction.

  Examples
- **We concentrated on** levels of patient satisfaction.
- **We studied** levels of patient satisfaction.

 Any of the verbs in **6. State research topic 1** can also be used in **7. State research topic 2**.

8. State the objectives 研究の目的を述べる

この研究の目的は，~です.

- **We wanted to see how** patients evaluated the products they used.

  Examples
- **Our objective was to find out** how patients reacted to different products.
- **The aim was to assess** the patients' evaluation of particular products.

40 Part 1 ● Starting 発表の始め方

9. Introduce the background 研究背景の説明を始める

それでは，はじめにこの研究の背景を説明します．

- I'd like to start with some background.

  Examples
- This is some background.
- Let's look at some background.
- I'll just run through some background.
- I'd like to show you some background.
- I'm going to show you the background.

発表内容の概略についての説明を終え，研究背景の説明に移るときは，左記のような表現を用いる．

 The word background is usually singular and always one word.
In the above examples, there are two expressions: some background and the background. Both are possible.

Background は単数形で用いることに注意する．また back ground と 2 単語に分割することはしない．some background と the background のいずれも用いることができる．

Key points

1. To save time, some presenters do not use an overview slide.
2. Instead, they give a short snapshot of the topic with no overview slide.
3. The material in 8. Pages 31〜41 can be used to create a short snapshot with no overview slide. Some functions can be omitted, depending on the structure of your presentation and the time available.

・目次スライドを使わずに発表を始めることもできる．

・その場合，発表のテーマや構成を口頭で簡単に紹介する．

9 Introduce the background
研究背景を紹介する

Presenters often include background information. This can vary from just a few sentences to several minutes of explanation with accompanying slides. In this section, I present key sentences for introducing background information.

> 発表テーマや発表の構成を説明した後は，研究背景の紹介に移る．

> 研究背景の紹介は，2,3文で終わらせる場合もあれば，数枚のスライドを用意してじっくりと説明する場合もある．

Script(研究背景を紹介するための原稿の例)

① This is some background. ② There has been a lot of work on improving memory or slowing down memory loss in old people. ③ Most studies have focused on light exercise as a way of reducing risk of dementia. ④ We know that light physical exercise such as gardening, mild stretching and slow walking for periods of about ten minutes increases connectivity between parts of the brain associated with making and storing memory. While these studies have used various types of light exercise, ⑤ no studies have focused on the effectiveness of individual types of exercise. ⑥ One of the main goals of this study was to compare the effectiveness of the following 5 types of exercise: mild stretching, gardening, slow walking, tai chi and cooking.

42　Part I ● Starting　発表の始め方

Key sentences

1. Introducing the background to your research
研究背景の紹介を始める

これからこの研究の背景についてご説明します.

■ **This is some background.**

Examples

■ **I'd like to start with** some background.

■ **I'd like to mention** the background of/to this study.

■ **I'd like to describe** the study background.

■ **I'm going to run through** some background.

■ **I want to go over** some background.

はじめに，研究背景の説明を始める合図として左記のように述べる.

The verbs **run through** and **go over** are used when you want to **focus only on the main points** and do not want to explain things in detail. The word **some** is usually used before **background**. Also, the word **background** in this context is **singular** and is one word. *Back ground* as two words is not correct.

詳細には踏み込まずに簡単に説明する，というニュアンスを伝えたいときは，句動詞 run through や go over を用いるとよい.（p. 57 のコラムも参照）

Background は単数形で，必ず1語として用いる. *Back ground* と2語に分割するのは誤り.

9 Introduce the background　研究背景を紹介する

2. Referring to known information　先行研究に言及する

～についてはこれまで多くの研究が行われてきました.

▌ <u>There has been a lot of work on</u> improving memory or slowing down memory loss in old people.

Examples

▌ <u>A lot of research has focused on</u> improving memory or slowing down memory loss in old people.

▌ As you know, <u>a lot of groups have been working on</u> improving memory or slowing down memory loss in old people.

▌ <u>There are several studies on</u> improving memory or slowing down memory loss in old people.

> **Note** In academic, written English, the above sentences would be as follows:
>
> ▌ Improving memory or slowing down memory loss in old people <u>has received a lot of attention</u>.
> ▌ Improving memory or slowing down memory loss in old people <u>has attracted a lot of attention</u>.
> ▌ A number of studies <u>have addressed the issue of</u> improving memory or slowing down memory loss in old people.

For an oral presentation, the patterns, **There has been a lot of work on / There are several studies on**, are more appropriate and easier to say.

まずは関連する先行研究について触れる.

先行研究について言及するとき, 論文などの書き言葉では左記のような表現となる. 話し言葉では, **There has been a lot of work on** や **There are several studies on** などの表現を用いるのが適切である.

44　Part I ● Starting　発表の始め方

3. Refer briefly to the studies mentioned in 2. Referring to known information
2で取り上げた研究の内容を簡単に紹介する

多くの研究は，〜について調べています.

▌ **Most studies have focused on** light exercise as a way of reducing risk of dementia.

Examples

▌ **Most of these studies have looked at** light exercise as a way of preventing memory loss.

▌ **The majority of studies have looked at** light exercise as a way of preventing memory loss.

▌ **The vast majority of studies have looked at** light exercise as a way of preventing memory loss.

This is an example of how to combine functions 1~3.

▌ Script(1～3をつなげた原稿の例)

I'd like to start with some background. There has been a lot of work on improving memory in people with mild dementia. Most studies have looked at light exercise as a way of preventing memory loss.

9 Introduce the background　研究背景を紹介する

4. What is known and currently accepted in the field
その研究領域で既に認められている考えを述べる

> 現在，〜ということが明らかになっています．

- **Currently, we know that** light exercise is a good way of preventing memory loss.

  Examples

- **We know that** light exercise is a good way of preventing memory loss.

 In academic, written English, the above sentence would be as follows:

- **It is known that** light exercise is a good way of preventing memory loss.
- **It is accepted that** light exercise is a good way of preventing memory loss.
- **It has been reported that** light exercise is a good way of preventing memory loss.

For an oral presentation, the patterns, **Currently, we know that** and **We know that**, are more appropriate and also easier to say.

研究の背景・目的の説明にあたっては，「先行研究によって○○が明らかになっている」→「しかし△△についてはまだよく分かっていない」→「そこで△△を明らかにするため，本研究を行った」という流れで説明するとよい．はじめに，**2, 3** で紹介した先行研究の結果，どのようなことが明らかになったのかを簡単に紹介する．

既知の情報を紹介するとき，論文などの書き言葉では左記のような表現を用いる．話し言葉では **Currently, we know that** や **We know that** と言う．

5. Research gap / niche 研究ギャップ／ニッチ

The expression **research gap / research niche** refers to an area of research or an issue that has received little or no attention.

続いて，どのような点がまだ分かっていないのか（研究ギャップ／ニッチ）を説明する．

しかし．～に注目した研究はありません．

- **No studies have focused on** the benefits of light exercise on memory.

  Examples

- **There has been no work on** the benefits of light exercise on memory.

- **Few studies have focused on** the benefits of light exercise on memory.

- **Studies on** the benefits of light exercise on memory **have been limited to** slow walking.

6. Research aims 研究の目的

It is important to state the aims of the study. In this case, the presenter mentions the aims at the end of the background. Aims can also be referred to as **goals**, **objectives** and **motivation**.

この研究は，～することを目的としています．

- **One of the main goals of this study was to** compare the effectiveness of the following 5 types of exercise: mild stretching, gardening, slow walking, tai chi and cooking.

9 Introduce the background 研究背景を紹介する

Examples are divided into 4 groups as follows: <u>goals</u>, <u>wanted</u>, <u>motivation</u> and <u>objectives</u>.

研究の目的を紹介する際は goals, wanted, motivation, objectives などの表現を活用する.

● Goals

▌ <u>One of the main goals of this study was to</u> assess the potential benefits of light exercise.

▌ <u>These were the goals of this study</u>: to assess the potential benefits of light exercise and to establish the most suitable forms of exercise.

▌ <u>One of our main goals was to</u> assess the potential benefits of light exercise.

▌ <u>One of our long-term goals was to</u> assess the potential benefits of light exercise.

▌ <u>Here are the goals</u>: to assess the potential benefits of light exercise and to establish the most suitable forms of exercise.

● Wanted

▌ <u>We wanted to look at</u> the potential benefits of light exercise.

▌ <u>We also wanted to look at</u> the differences between the effectiveness of exercise types.

● Motivation

▌ <u>The main motivation of this study was to</u> assess the potential benefits of light exercise.

● Objective

▌ <u>Our principle objective was to</u> assess the potential benefits of light exercise.

▌ <u>Our main objective was to</u> assess the potential benefits of light exercise.

▌ <u>The objective of this study was to</u> assess the potential benefits of light exercise.

10 How to start a presentation as an invited speaker
招待講演の始め方

In this section, I introduce some useful sentences to use as an invited speaker.

Here is an example.

Script(招待講演を開始するときの原稿例)

① Thank you very much for the introduction. ② Before I start, I'd like to say a big thank you to the organizers for inviting me. It is indeed a great honor to be here.

③ As you probably know, I'm a materials engineer. Currently, I'm at Imperial College, London in the Department of Engineering. ④ We are doing research on metal fatigue. ⑤ We are also interested in failure in other materials. ⑥ In recent years, we have been focusing on self-healing materials. ⑦ I'd like to start by giving a brief introduction to our work.

Key sentences

1. Thanking the chairperson　座長へのお礼

ご紹介ありがとうございます.

▌ **Thank you very much for the introduction.**

　Examples

▌ **Thank you,** Dr. Watanabe, **for introducing me.**

▌ **Thank you, Professor Williams, for that nice introduction. And thanks also to the rest of the committee for inviting me.**

▌ **Thanks, Bill, for introducing me.**

通常の口頭発表と同様, 最初は座長へのお礼を述べる.

2. Thanking the organizers　学会主催者，実行委員へのお礼

このような機会をいただけたことに感謝いたします.

■ **Before I start, I'd like to say a big thank you to** the organizers for inviting me.

Examples

■ **I'd like to say that it is a great pleasure and an honor to be invited to speak here today**.

■ **I must say that it is a great honor to present at this conference. I would very much like to thank the organizers, particularly Dr. Suzuki from Tokyo University, who has made all the arrangements for my trip**.

■ **Thank you very much indeed for this kind invitation. It is indeed a great honor to be here**.

■ **Thank you very much for giving me the opportunity to speak at this conference**.

座長へのお礼に続いて，学会の主催者や実行委員に対し，招待講演の場を設けてくれたことへのお礼を述べる.

3. Background　所属，研究領域などの紹介

〜の分野で研究しています.

■ **As you probably know, I'm a materials engineer**.

Examples

■ **I'm a materials engineer**.

■ **My background is in** materials engineering.

■ **I have a background in** materials engineering.

■ **I'd just like to mention my background and current research**.

■ **I'm a** medical doctor and **have a background in** community health.

■ **Basically, I am an environmental engineer. My main interest is in building materials. In other words, composite materials used in construction. For example, concrete**.

自己紹介として，職業・所属や研究領域などについて説明する.

50　Part I ● Starting　発表の始め方

- So, I'm at Imperial College, London in the Department of Engineering. As you probably know, we are working on self-healing construction materials, particularly concrete.
- Currently, I'm at Imperial College, London in the Department of Engineering.

4. Research interests 1 研究内容の説明（1）

主に〜について調べています.

- We are doing research on metal fatigue.

Examples

- My main research interest is metal fatigue.
- Our main research focus is on metal fatigue.

4〜6 では，通常の口頭発表と同様に，自分がどのような研究を行っているかを簡単に説明する.

5. Research interests 2 研究内容の説明（2）

また，〜についても調べています.

- We are also interested in failure in other materials.

6. Current research 現在の研究課題の紹介

最近は，主に〜のテーマについて研究を進めています.

- In recent years, we have been focusing on self-healing materials.

Examples

- Right now, we are working on (topic).

7. Starting 講演の開始

それでは，はじめに〜についてお話しします．

■ **I'd like to start by giving a brief introduction to our work.**

Examples

■ **I'll start by talking about** (topic).

■ **I'd like to start with some background.**

■ **I'll spend the first 5 minutes of my presentation talking about** (topic).

挨拶，自己紹介を終えて講演の本題に入るときは，左記のように言う．

11 Useful sentences for: Thanking the audience for coming, Making informal opening comments, Giving a series of talks, Comments when you present after a well-known presenter, Dealing with technical problems　便利な表現集

In this section, I include a variety of useful sentences that do not fit in the categories already covered in this section.

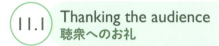

11.1　Thanking the audience
聴衆へのお礼

At conferences where there are multiple, simultaneous sessions, some presenters start by thanking the audience for attending. Here are some examples.

1. Thanking people for coming to your presentation
   自分の発表を聴きに来てくれたことへのお礼

- Thank you for coming today.
- Thank you very much for coming today.
- Before I start, I'd just like to say thank you for coming today.

2. Thanking attendees for attending a session scheduled late in the day or at the end of a conference　最終演題や最終日に聴きに来てくれたことへのお礼

- This is the last presentation slot today. So, thank you very much for coming.
- It's the last day of the conference. I'd like to thank you for sticking around and coming to this presentation.
- This is the last day of the conference and also the last session. I must say that I'm very pleased to see so many people. Thank you for coming.

11.2 Informal opening comments
発表開始時に用いるくだけた挨拶表現

At an informal presentation, you may want to make some opening comments.

▎ **It's great to see so many people here**. **Thank you for coming**.

▎ There are just a few people here today, **so please feel free to ask questions whenever you like**.

11.3 Useful sentences for when you are giving a series of talks
複数回にわたって講演する際に用いる表現

If you are giving a series of talks over a number of days or weeks, possibly as a visiting professor, or several presentations at the same conference, the following sentences may be useful.

1. Refer to previous presentations 前回のおさらい

▎ **My last talk focused on** theoretical approaches. **This evening I'll be talking about** applications and our ongoing research work.

▎ **Previously, I spoke about** self-healing materials, particularly paint. **Today, I want to talk about** (topic).

▎ **Last week, I spoke about / focused on** self-healing materials, particularly paint. **This presentation is on** (topic).

▎ **So, in my last lecture I was talking about** self-healing materials, particularly paint. **Today, I will be covering** (topic).

▎ I can see some people here who were at my presentation in Korea last week. **I'd just like to say that I'm going to cover some of the same ground, but I'll also be focusing on pain and the temporomandibular joint**. **So, you will have heard some of this before**, **but the majority of what I have to say is new**.

54　Part I ● Starting　発表の始め方

2. Refer to future presentations 次回の講演内容の予告

- **I'd just like to mention that I have one more presentation on** Tuesday. It's on (topic). **If you are interested, please come along. It would be great to see you.**
- **I have one more talk next week, which will be on** (topic). That will be my last talk.
- **Next week, I'll be talking about** (topic).
- **I'll be covering** (topic) **in the next presentation, which is on Friday.**

11.4 Comments when you present after a well-known presenter
著名な演者のすぐ後に発表する場合のコメント

In some cases, you will need to present after a well-known presenter. Here are some useful sentences that are divided into 2 steps. In step 1, you can make a short comment on the previous presentation. In step 2, you start your presentation.

Step 1 前の演者の発表に言及する

- **It is a difficult task to speak after** Dr Williams' wonderful presentation.
- **It is not easy to speak after** such an impressive presentation.
- **I think that Dr. Williams has just about said everything there is to say about** (topic).
- **After Dr. Williams' wonderful presentation, there is not much left for me to say.**

Step 2 自分の発表を始める

- However, I have some recent data that I hope will be of interest to you. So, I'd like to get started.
- However, it is possible that some of the material I'm covering today will fit in nicely with Dr Williams' presentation.

Useful sentences for: Thanking the audience for coming, Making informal opening comments, Giving a series of talks, Comments when you present after a well-known presenter, Dealing with technical problems　便利な表現集

11.5 Dealing with technical problems
PC, プロジェクターなどに問題が起こった場合の対応

Most presenters will have experienced some kind of technical problems with computers, projectors and so on. Here are some useful sentences to use in those situations.

1. Apologizing for a technical problem at the beginning of the presentation
発表の最初にトラブルが起こった場合

▌ <u>Sorry about the</u> technical problems.

▌ <u>I'm afraid we are having some technical problems</u>.

▌ <u>I'm afraid we are having some problems with</u> this computer / system / projector.

2. After the problem has been solved　トラブル解決後の一言

▌ <u>Sorry to have kept you waiting</u>.

▌ <u>I think we can get started now</u>.

▌ <u>Ok. I think we are ready to start now</u>.

3. Apologizing for problems that occur in the middle of the presentation
発表の途中にトラブルが起こった場合

Sometimes problems may occur **in the middle of your presentation**. Here are some useful sentences.

▌ <u>Sorry about that. I had an issue with some software / this computer / a video clip</u>.

▌ <u>We are having problems with the connection. Just a moment. Okay, we have fixed that. I'd like to continue</u>.

56　Part 1 ● Starting　発表の始め方

4. When something such as a video clip or animation does not work
映像が流れない，アニメーションが動かないなどのトラブル

▌ **We're having trouble with** the computer / the sound system / an adaptor.

▌ **There's an issue with** the computer / the sound system / an adaptor.

▌ **I had hoped to** show you a video clip. **But that doesn't seem to be possible. I'd like to move on to** the next section.

▌ **I had a brief video clip I wanted to show you,** but it doesn't seem to be working. **So I'll skip that.**

▌ **I wanted to show you** a video clip of the reaction, **but I have had a technical issue.**

▌ **I'll have to skip the video. Sorry about that.** / **I apologize for that.**

Column #02

I'll just run through / go over the main points
Run through，go over を上手に使おう

The expressions **run through** and **go over** signal to the audience that you will <u>concentrate on the most important information on a slide</u>.

▌ I'll just run through the main points.

▌ There is a lot of data here. I'll run through the most important results.

▌ I'll just go over the important data.

▌ There is a lot of data here. I'll go over the main points.

It is highly likely that some of your slides are going to be busy and, on some occasions, you will have to skip some material. This is exactly when the expressions **run through** and **go over** will be useful.

「詳細には触れず，本当に重要なポイントだけを簡単に説明します」と言いたいときは，run through や go over という表現が最適である．

Useful sentences for: Thanking the audience for coming, Making informal opening comments, Giving a series of talks, Comments when you present after a well-known presenter, Dealing with technical problems　便利な表現集

Part 2
Using informal, spoken English to simplify and shorten the main body
話し言葉の英語を活用して簡潔な原稿を作成する方法

In this section, I provide examples of **how to change formal English to informal English**. Each example has a formal sentence and examples in informal English.

　口頭発表で使われる「話し言葉」の英語は，論文で使われる「書き言葉」の英語とは異なります．口頭発表の原稿に論文の文章をそのままもってくると，口頭で読み上げるには不向きな，長く堅苦しい表現ばかりになってしまいます．この章では多数の例をもとに，論文調の書き言葉の英語を話し言葉の英語に変換する方法を紹介します．

I How to reduce the level of formality in your presentation
書き言葉の英語を話し言葉の英語に変換する方法

Note The example sentences presented in this section are for oral presentations and are generally too informal for use in an academic paper.

本章で紹介する例文はいずれも口頭発表用のものであり，論文で使用するのは適切でないことに注意してほしい．

Let's start by looking at a typical example of written academic English.

以下，書き言葉の文章をグレーの四角の中に，話し言葉の英語に直した例文を緑色の四角の中に示す．

▪ The receptor <u>has been shown to play</u> an important role in the mechanism.

1. <u>We know that</u> the receptor <u>has</u> an important role in the mechanism.
2. <u>The receptor has</u> an important role in the mechanism.
3. <u>The receptor is</u> important <u>in terms of</u> the mechanism.

元の文章は受動態であるが，1〜3 ではすべて能動態となっている．

「〜について」「〜において」と言いたいときは，3 のように in terms of を用いるとよい．

Here are some examples of how to reduce the formality of this sentence.
You will notice that example 1 starts with **we** and is **active** not **passive**. The verb **shown to play** has been deleted. Examples 2 and 3 are also in the active tense. Sentence 3 uses the useful expression **in terms of**. Examples 1 〜 3 are much shorter and less formal than the original.

Part 2 ● Using informal, spoken English to simplify and shorten the main body
話し言葉の英語を活用して簡潔な原稿を作成する方法

■ This lipid is expected to be used as a detergent and a lubricant.

1. **We think that** this lipid can be used as a detergent or lubricant.
2. **This lipid can probably be used as** a detergent or lubricant.

	1 は is expected to を We think that で置き換えている.
	2 は probably を用いることで確信の度合いを弱めた表現にしている.

The formality has been reduced by changing the expression **is expected to** to **we think that**. In example 2, the strength of the statement has been reduced by using the expression **can probably be used as**.

■ These systems are expected to have applications in the medical field.

1. **We think** these systems have medical applications.
2. **These systems have** medical applications.

Example 1 is an active sentence starting with **we**, using the word **think** instead of **expected**. In example 2, **we think** has been omitted. **These systems have** medical applications. Example 2 is more direct and stronger in tone than **These systems are expected to have applications in the medical field**. The original sentence has eleven words. Example 2 has only five words. The original sentence is too formal for an oral presentation.

元の文章は受動態であるが, 1 は We think で始まる能動態の文となっている.

2 のように, We think を削除して確信の度合いを高めた表現にすることもできる.

このように話し言葉に変換することで, 語数を元の文章の 11 語から, 1 では 7 語, 2 では 5 語にまで減らすことができ, 時間の限られた口頭発表の場でも読み上げやすくなる.

How to reduce the level of formality in your presentation
書き言葉の英語を話し言葉の英語に変換する方法

■ It is suggested that the difference is caused by plastic deformation.

1. **We think that the difference is caused** by plastic deformation.
2. **This difference is caused by** plastic deformation.
3. **The difference is due to** plastic deformation.
4. **The difference is probably caused by** plastic deformation.

The phrase **It is suggested that** has been deleted because it is too formal for a presentation. The meaning of **It is suggested** is expressed by the phrases **We think that** or **The difference is probably caused by**. The word **probably** in example 4 is used to **tone down the strength of the sentence**.

> **Note** The phrase **It is suggested that** is weaker than **The difference is due to**.
> In an oral presentation, it is acceptable to use strong statements such as **the difference is due to**. In a written paper, however, it might be necessary to **tone down the strength of your statement** by using expressions like **It is suggested that / It is thought that / It is considered that**. While these expressions are used in written English, they are not commonly used in oral presentations.

It is suggested は論文的な表現なので削除する．

It is suggested のように確信の度合いを弱める表現を残したい場合は，1, 4 のように We think や probably を用いる．確信の度合いを上げた表現とする場合は，2, 3 のように言い切ってしまえばよい．

口頭発表では通常，論文とは異なり断定的な表現を用いてもよい．一方論文では，断定できるだけの根拠がない場合には It is suggested that, It is thought that, It is considered that などの確信の度合いを下げる表現を用いる必要がある．

■ From the present data, <u>it is thought that</u> reliability increases by about 20 percent.

1. <u>**As the data shows, there is an increase in**</u> reliability of about 20 percent.
2. <u>**As the data shows, reliability increases by about**</u> 20 percent.
3. <u>**These results/data indicate**</u> that there is an increase in reliability of about 20 percent.
4. <u>**These results/data show an increase in**</u> reliability of about 20 percent.
5. <u>**There is an increase in**</u> reliability of about 20 percent.
6. <u>**So, this means that**</u> there is an increase in reliability of about 20 percent.

The phrase **from the present data** has been deleted because it is unnecessary. The expression, **it is thought that** has also been deleted. In example 6, the phrase **So, this means that** refers to the data that has been presented. The shortest sentence is 5., which uses the simple pattern, <u>**There is an increase in**</u> reliability of about 20 percent. Please note the preposition <u>**in**</u> after the word increase.

■ Earthquakes <u>are categorized into</u> 3 types.

1. <u>**There are 3 types of**</u> earthquakes.

The sentence pattern has been changed and the word **categorized** deleted. Example 1 starts with **there**. The revised sentence is much easier to say.

「お示ししたデータから〜ということが分かります」と言いたいとき，論文では from the present data を用いるが，口頭発表ではより簡単に As the data shows, や The results/data indicate, So, this means that などとする。

「データから〜」の部分を省略し，5 のように言ってもよい。

Increase の後ろにくる前置詞は in であることに注意する。

「〜種類に分類される」は「〜つの種類がある」と言い換えられる。Categorized を削除し，より簡単な文にすることで発音もしやすくなる。

How to reduce the level of formality in your presentation
書き言葉の英語を話し言葉の英語に変換する方法

■ It is <u>anticipated / expected / predicted / thought / suggested</u> that the intensity of typhoons will increase in the future.

1. <u>We think that</u> the intensity of typhoons will increase in the future.
2. <u>This data suggests that</u> typhoons will become stronger in the future.
3. <u>Typhoons will probably increase</u> in intensity in the future.
4. <u>It is quite likely / highly likely</u> that typhoons will increase in intensity in the future.
5. <u>We think that</u> typhoons will get stronger.

It is anticipated / expected / predicted / thought / suggested はいずれも論文的な表現なので，口頭発表では避けたほうがよい．

4 では，quite likely, highly likely を用いることで，確信の度合いを高めた表現としている．

5 では，increase in intensity（強度が増す）を get stronger と言い換えている．

The verbs **anticipated**, **expected**, **predicted**, **thought**, **suggested** have been deleted as they are more suitable for academic papers. Example 1 is active and uses the phrase **We think that**. Example 3 uses simple grammar: **Typhoons will probably increase in intensity in the future**. In example 4, the strength of the sentence can be varied by using the expressions **quite likely**, **highly likely**. Sentence 5 is the shortest and only has seven words. **Get stronger** is an informal expression that means **increase in intensity**.

> Note It is better to avoid sentences patterns like these in your presentations: **It is anticipated / expected / predicted / thought / concluded / suggested that**. These expressions are more suitable for written English.

■ The device does not have any faults.

1. The device <u>has no faults</u>.
2. <u>There are no faults</u>.

In this example, it is possible to reduce the number of words from seven to four.

元の文章は「欠陥がない」を does not have any faults で表しているが，これを has no faults や There are no faults に置き換えることで，語数を減らすことができる．

■ It has been reported that online interventions in the form of questionnaires and reminders can help at risk people to control their weight.

1. **We know that** online interventions in the form of questionnaires and reminders can help people to control their weight.

> It has been reported that は論文中で既知の情報に触れる際によく使われる表現であるが, 口頭発表ではより簡潔に We know that とするとよい.

The expression **It has been reported that** is commonly found in written academic English. In oral presentations, a short, simple expression is **We know that**.
See page 38 for more information on how to refer to other data.

■ We succeeded in fabricating new materials.

1. **We were able to make** new materials.
2. **We were able to produce** new materials.
3. **We managed to make** new materials.
4. **We managed to produce** new materials.
5. **We made** new materials.
6. **We produced** new materials.

> 「〜することに成功した」を succeeded in 〜 ing とするのは論文的な堅苦しい表現である. 話し言葉では,「なんとか成し遂げた」というニュアンスを含めたい場合は managed to (+ make/produce) を用い, その必要がない場合は 5, 6 のように単に「〜した」という形にする.

The expression **succeeded in fabricating** is quite formal and grammatically complex. It stresses the difficulty of doing something. Here are some examples with easier expressions using **were able to**, **managed to**, **made**, **produced**.
The simplest sentences are as follows: **We made** and **We produced**. Unless there is a specific need to stress that production was difficult to achieve, it is better to use **made** or **produced** in the simple past tense than **we succeeded in + verb + ing**.

- Epicenters have received a lot of attention.
- Epicenters have attracted a lot of attention.

The expressions **have received a lot of attention / have attracted a lot of attention** are commonly found in the introduction sections of academic papers. Here are some less formal examples commonly used in oral presentations.

1. A lot of people are working on epicenters.
2. A lot of people are doing research on epicenters.
3. A lot of people are focusing on epicenters.
4. There has been a lot of research on epicenters.
5. There has been a lot of work on epicenters.
6. Epicenters are an important topic.
7. Epicenters are a hot topic.

In examples 1-3, the informal verbs **work on**, **do research on**, **focus on** are used. In examples 4 and 5, the words **research** and **work** are nouns that take the preposition **on**. Common patterns are **a lot of research on** and **a lot of work on**. Examples 6 and 7 use the verb are in the patterns, **are an important topic**, **are a hot topic**.

先行研究について「〜についての研究は多い」と言いたいとき，論文では have received a lot of attention, have attracted a lot of attention と受動態の文章とするが，口頭発表では「多くの人が〜について研究している」(1〜3)，「〜についての研究は多い」(4, 5)，「〜は注目のテーマである」(6, 7) のように能動態で表現する。

1〜3 では，話し言葉でよく使われる句動詞 work on, do research on, focus on を用いている。

4, 5 では，research, work を名詞として用いている．後に続く前置詞は両方とも on であることに注意する．

6, 7 は，注目のテーマであることを are an important topic, are a hot topic という表現で示している．

■ In the literature, there are few reports on adhesives suitable for this kind of restoration.

1. There <u>are few reports on</u> adhesives suitable for this kind of restoration.
2. <u>No studies have focused on</u> adhesives suitable for this kind of restoration.
3. There <u>is not much data on</u> adhesives suitable for this kind of restoration.
4. There are <u>few people working on</u> adhesives suitable for this kind of restoration.
5. <u>Few people are working on</u> adhesives suitable for this kind of restoration.
6. There <u>has not been much work on</u> adhesives suitable for this kind of restoration.
7. There <u>has not been any work on</u> adhesives suitable for this kind of restoration.

The above sentence, **In the literature, there are few reports on** (topic) is grammatically correct, but the use of the expression **in the literature** makes it quite formal. The examples 1〜7 show simpler sentences with the same meaning that do not use **in the literature**. For examples of how to use the expression **in the literature** correctly, please see page 166.

前ページの例とは逆に「〜についての研究は少ない」と言いたいときは左記のように言う.

In the literature という表現は論的な印象を与えるので使用を避ける. 正しい使い方については p. 166 を参照.

How to reduce the level of formality in your presentation
書き言葉の英語を話し言葉の英語に変換する方法

■ Candidates <u>were assigned</u> to 3 groups.

1. <u>We divided</u> candidates <u>into</u> 3 groups.
2. <u>We put</u> candidates <u>into</u> 3 groups.
3. <u>We assigned</u> candidates <u>to</u> 3 groups.

The sentence has been changed from passive to active. In examples 1 and 2, the formal verb **assigned** has been changed to **divided into** or **put into**. **Assigned** is the most formal verb and **put** is the most informal verb. Assigned is used in example 3 in an active sentence.

「対象者を○群に割り当てた」と言いたいとき，assign を受動態で用いるのは論文的な表現なので，話し言葉では We divided〜into〜groups や We put〜into〜groups とする。Assign を用いる場合も能動態で用いる。

■ Novel devices <u>are being intensively studied</u> to solve the problem of energy consumption.

1. **A lot of people are <u>working on</u>** new devices to solve the problem of energy consumption.
2. **A lot of people are <u>looking at</u>** new devices to solve the problem of energy consumption.
3. **A lot of people are <u>doing research on</u>** new devices to solve the problem of energy consumption.
4. <u>Several groups</u> are <u>doing research on</u> new devices to solve the problem of energy consumption.
5. <u>Many researchers are working on</u> new devices to solve the problem of energy consumption.

The original sentence looks as if it has been copied from the introduction of an academic paper. It is too formal for an oral presentation. The verb **studied** has been changed to **working on**, **looking at**, and **doing research on**. The examples are active.

「〜は集中的に研究されている」(are being intensively studied) は論文的な表現なので，「多くの人が〜について研究している」と言い換え，能動態の現在進行形の文にするとよい。「研究する」を表す動詞も，study ではなく work on, look at, do research on などを用いる。

■ These results strongly suggest that adhesion is at lower levels than previously reported.

1. **So, this means that** adhesion is at lower levels **than previously reported**.
2. **This means that** adhesion is at lower levels **than previously reported.**
3. **Adhesion is at** lower levels **than previously reported**.
4. **Adhesion is at** lower levels **than we previously thought**.
5. **Adhesion is at** lower levels **than we thought**.

「この結果は〜」と言いたいときは，話し言葉では (So) this means that とするとよい．3〜5のように，この部分を省略してさらに簡潔に述べることもできる．

「以前報告されていたよりも」「以前考えられていたよりも」と言いたいときは，than previously reported よりも口語的な表現として than we (previously) thought とすることもできる．

The expression **These results strongly suggest that** is formal. Examples 1 and 2 use less formal expressions, **So this means that** and **This means that**, both of which refer to the results that have just been presented. The sentence can be shortened by deleting **These results strongly suggest that**. In examples 4 and 5, **than previously reported** has been changed to more informal expressions **than we previously thought** and **than we thought**. Example 5 has eight words whereas the original sentence has thirteen.

■ The system is under development.

1. **The system is being developed**.
2. **We are (currently) developing** the system.
3. **We are (currently) working on** the system.

元の文章では「〜は開発中である」を under development としているが，1〜3 はいずれも現在進行形で表現している．2, 3 の currently は省略しても構わない．

In examples 2 and 3, the word **we** is used with the verbs **developing** and **working on**. If necessary, the word **currently** can be deleted.

■ From these results, it was concluded that reliability increased.

1. **These results show** that reliability increased.
2. **As you can see,** reliability increased.
3. **Reliability increased.**

> 「この結果から，〜のように結論づけられる」は論文では From these results, it was concluded となるが，話し言葉では 1〜3 のように簡潔に述べるとよい．

The expression **it was concluded that** is commonly found in academic papers and is too formal for oral presentations. The three examples are much simpler, shorter and easier to say. They have been changed from passive to active. The expression **from these results** is unnecessary and has been deleted.

■ A significant increase in values was observed in group 1.

1. **We found that** values increased significantly in group 1.
2. **There was a** significant increase in values in group 1.
3. **Values increased** significantly in group 1.
4. **Values increased a lot** in group 1.
5. **Group 1 values** increased a lot.

> 「〜が観察された／みられた」は論文では受動態で was observed となるが，話し言葉では We found や There was のように能動態とする．また，この部分を省略して 3〜5 のようにさらに簡潔な文にすることもできる．

The sentence has been changed from passive to active and starts with **we found** or **there was**. It is also possible to omit **we found** and **there was**, and start the sentence with the word **values**. For example, 3. **Values increased significantly in group 1** and 4. **Values increased a lot in group 1**. Example 5, **Group 1 values increased a lot** is the shortest.

▍Furthermore, reliability was analyzed.

1. **We also looked at** reliability.
2. **We also focused on** reliability.
3. **We also analyzed** reliability.
4. **In addition, we analyzed** reliability.

Furthermore, reliability was analyzed is an example of written scientific English using the passive and a formal verb **analyzed**. The sentence has been changed from passive to active, and the word **furthermore** has been changed to **also** or **in addition**. The informal two-word verbs **look at** and **focus on** have been used instead of the more formal **was analyzed**. In examples 3 and 4, **analyzed** is used in an active sentence using **we**.

「〜について調べた」と言うとき，**analyze** を受動態で用いると論文的な表現になるので，話し言葉では能動態として，また **look at** や **focus on** などの句動詞を用いるとよい．

「さらに〜」は **furthermore** よりも **also** や **in addition** のほうが話し言葉に適した表現である．

▍In the present study, a new simulation method was employed.

1. **We used** a new simulation method.
2. A new simulation method **was used**.

The expression **in the present study** is redundant and should be deleted because it is obvious that you are talking about your current research and not some other research. The word **employed** has been changed to **used**. The expression **in the present study** is generally only used when you are talking about a series of studies and relating them to each other. Example 1 is active and example 2 is passive.

「この研究では〜という手法を用いた」と言うとき，「この研究では」（**in the present study**）の部分はわざわざ言及しなくとも明らかであり，口頭発表では省略する．また「（手法を）用いる」の動詞は論文では **employ** となるが，口頭発表ではより平易な **use** とする．

■ The level must not <u>be in excess of</u> 20 percent.
■ The level must <u>not exceed</u> 20 percent.

1. The level <u>must not be more than</u> 20 percent.
2. The level <u>should not be more than</u> 20 percent.

「超過する」は論文では **be in excess of** や **exceed** が用いられるが，話し言葉では **be more than** とするとよい。

The formality of the expressions **must not be in excess of** and **must not exceed** should be reduced. **In excess of** and **exceed** can be changed to **must not be more than** or **should not be more than**.

■ The system <u>can be applied in a variety of industries</u> such as construction.

1. <u>We can use</u> this system in industries such as construction.
2. <u>You can use</u> this system in industries such as construction.
3. <u>This system can be used in</u> industries such as construction.
4. <u>This system can be used in</u> construction.

元の文章は受動態で **can be applied** となっているが，1, 2 では **We (You) can use** で始まる能動態の文になっている。この場合，**We** でも **You** でもどちらでもよい。

1〜4 とも，元の文章の **a variety of** を省略して語数を減らしている。4 はさらに **industries such as** も省いている。

In examples 1 and 2, the sentence structure has been changed from passive to active. The word **applied** has been changed to **you can use**. Please note that **you** and **we** can both be used. In the last example, <u>industries such as</u> has been deleted and the sentence starts with the expression: <u>This system can be used in</u> (construction).

> ▌The mechanism has not been elucidated.
> ▌The mechanism is unknown.
> ▌The mechanism is not fully understood.

The above three sentences have the same meaning. Sentence 1 is the most formal because it uses the word **elucidate**.

1. **We do not know anything about** the mechanism.
2. **We do not know much about** the mechanism.
3. **There is not much data on** the mechanism.
4. **There is no data on** the mechanism.
5. **We are still working on** the mechanism.
6. **We are still studying** the mechanism.
7. **We are still analyzing** the mechanism.

Example 1 is active and starts with the expression **we do not know**. The expression **is not fully understood** has been changed to **we do not know anything about / much about**. Example 5 uses the two-word verb **working on**, which has the same meaning as **studying** or **analyzing**. The sentence, **We are still working on the mechanism** is another way of saying **The mechanism is not fully understood**. The word **elucidated** **is too formal for an oral presentation**. Its frequency is low and mostly restricted to academic papers.

「～については分かっていない」と言いたいときは，「私達は～については知らない」(1, 2)，「～についてのデータはない」(3, 4)，「私達は～については研究中である」(5～7) のいずれかの形で述べるとよい．

動詞 elucidate は堅苦しい表現であり，学術論文では使用されるが，口頭発表では通常用いられない．

① How to reduce the level of formality in your presentation
書き言葉の英語を話し言葉の英語に変換する方法

▌This issue <u>has been addressed</u> by a lot of / by many / by a number of theoretical chemists.

1. A lot of theoretical chemists <u>are looking at</u> this problem/issue.
2. A lot of theoretical chemists <u>are working on</u> this problem/issue.
3. A lot of theoretical chemists <u>are doing research on</u> this problem/issue.
4. A lot of theoretical chemists <u>are studying</u> this problem/issue.

「～については多くの研究が行われてきた」は「多くの研究者が～について研究している」と能動態の文に直すとよい。その際，「研究する」を表す動詞は **looking at**, **working on**, **doing research on**, **studying** などとする。

This sentence has been changed from passive to active. In order to reduce formality, I have changed the formal verb **address** to <u>**looking at**</u>, <u>**working on**</u>, <u>**doing research on**</u>, <u>**studying**</u>.

(Note) The expression, *we are studying on*, is incorrect. The preposition **on** can be used in the following patterns: **This is <u>a study on</u> reliability. We carried out <u>a study on</u> reliability.** In both of the examples, the word **study** is a noun and is followed by the preposition **on**. The word **study** has two patterns.
1. To study + topic (this is a verb) Example, **A lot of theoretical chemists <u>are studying</u> this problem**.
2. A study on + topic (this is a noun) Example, **We <u>did a study on</u> rates of biodegradability**.

Study の後に前置詞 **on** をつけるかどうかは，**study** を動詞として用いているか名詞として用いているかによって異なる。動詞の場合，**study** は他動詞なので **on** はつけない（**We study + topic**）。名詞の場合は前置詞 **on** が必要となる（**a study on + topic**）。

■ The apparatus is equipped with a temperature gauge.

1. **There is a** temperature gauge.
2. **The apparatus has a** temperature gauge.
3. **The apparatus consists of a** temperature gauge, (a) microcomputer and (a) monitor.

You can reduce the formality of this sentence by deleting **equipped with**. The sentence has been simplified by deleting the expression **equipped with** and using the verbs **is**, **has** and **consists of**. If the apparatus has a number of functions, you can use **consists of** and a simple list of components as in example 3.

「装置には温度計を搭載している」は論文では be equipped with を用いた受動態の文章になるが，口頭発表では is や has を用いた能動態の文にする．また装置の構成を述べる際は，3 のように consists of の後に続けて構成要素を簡単に列挙してもよい．

■ It is possible to purchase an SD card whose capacity is in excess of 40 GB.
■ It is possible to purchase an SD card the capacity of which is in excess of 40 GB.

1. You can buy an SD card that **has over** 40 GB.
2. You can buy an SD card that **has capacity over** 40 GB.
3. You can buy an SD card **with capacity over** 40 GB.

It is possible → You can
purchase → buy
is in excess of → over

The phrases **whose capacity is in excess of** and **the capacity of which is in excess of** are usually used in written scientific English. They have been deleted and the new sentence pattern starts with the word **you**. The word **purchased** has been changed to **buy**. The expression **whose capacity is in excess of 40 GB** has been changed to **has over 40 GB**.

① How to reduce the level of formality in your presentation
書き言葉の英語を話し言葉の英語に変換する方法

■ We <u>adopted</u> a new system.

1. <u>We used</u> a new system.
2. <u>We chose</u> a new system.
3. <u>We employed</u> a new system.

The word **adopted** has been changed to, **used**, **chose**, **employed**. **Use** and **employ** have the same meaning, but **employ** is a lot more formal.

> 動詞 adopt の代わりに use, choose, employ を用いている。Use と employ はほぼ同じ意味であるが，employ はやや堅苦しい表現である．

■ Differences in performance <u>were observed</u>.
■ Differences in performance <u>were noted</u>.
■ Differences in performance <u>were seen</u>.

1. <u>There were</u> differences in performance.
2. <u>There were</u> variations in performance.
3. <u>Performance varied</u>.
4. <u>We observed</u> differences in performance.
5. <u>We noted</u> differences in performance.
6. <u>We saw</u> differences in performance.

In the first three examples, the verbs **observed**, **noted** and **seen** are not used.
Example 3 is the shortest and easiest to say. <u>Performance varied</u>.
In examples 4〜6, the verbs **observed**, **noted** and **saw** are used in active sentences.

> 「〜が観察された」「〜がみられた」は受動態で論文的な表現なので，話し言葉では「〜があった」(1, 2) や「私達は〜を観察した」(4〜6) のように言う．

> 「〜の差が観察された」を「〜が変化した」と言い換えることで，3 のようにより簡潔に表現することもできる．

▌Here we have the experimental setup. Its length is 14 meters.

1. The experimental setup is 14 meters in length.
2. The setup is 14 meters in length.
3. The setup is 14 meters long.
4. The setup is 14 meters.

There is a big difference in the formality of the sentences **Here we have the experimental setup** and **Its length is 14 meters**. The first, **Here we have the experimental setup**, is informal and the second, **Its length is 14 meters**, is formal and mostly restricted to written scientific usage. The 4 example sentences are less formal. The most informal sentence is the last one. **The setup is 14 meters**.

> 元の文章は前半は口語的な表現であるが、後半は論文的な表現になってしまっている。「長さは〜メートルである」と言いたいとき、話し言葉では左記の1〜4のように表現する。

▌Another experiment was performed.
▌Another experiment was carried out.

1. **We did** another experiment.

The verbs **performed** and **carried out** are formal and mostly used in written English.
The verb **did** is informal and easier to use. You can repeat the verb **do** several times. This is quite normal in an oral presentation. For example: **We did an experiment on** X. **We also did several experiments on** Y. **The next day, we did a follow-up experiment**. In this case, the word **did** is used three times. Repetition of verbs such as **do** and **look at** is not a problem in an oral presentation.

> 「実験を行った」は論文では performed や carried out を用いて受動態で表現するが、口頭発表ではより単純に We did で表すとよい。

> 左記の例では動詞 do を3連続で使用しているが、do や look at を何度も繰り返し用いるのは口頭発表では問題ない。

▌Data was obtained from several different locations.

1. **We gathered** data from several different locations.
2. **We collected** data from several different locations.
3. **We took** data from several different locations.
4. **We got** data from several different locations.

「データを収集した」を obtained よりも平易な動詞 gathered, collected, took, got で表している（got は get の過去形）。

The verb **obtained** has been changed to **gathered**, **collected**, **took**, **got**. The example sentences are all active. The most informal verb is **got**. Please note that **got** is the past tense of **get**.

▌It can be classified into 2 types.
▌It can be divided into 2 types.

1. **There are 2 types.**

「○つのタイプに分類される」(be classified into 〜 types) は「○つのタイプがある」(There are 〜 types) と言い換えることができる。

The verbs **classified into** and **divided into** have been deleted. The sentence has been reduced to four words. The simple pattern, **There is/are**, is a useful pattern for oral presentations.

この例のように、There is/are を用いて端的に状態を表した文は、口頭発表では非常に有用である。

▌This is an image of the electric power flow.

1. <u>Here you can see</u> the electric power flow.
2. <u>You can see</u> the electric power flow <u>here</u>.
3. <u>This is</u> the electric power flow.
4. <u>This shows</u> the electric power flow.
5. <u>Here we have</u> the electric power flow.

The word **image** has been deleted in order to shorten the sentence and make it easier to say. The sentence has been reduced from nine words to six. **This is the electric power flow**.

スライド内の図を示して「これは〜を示した図です」(**This is an image of**)と言いたいとき，「を示した図」(**an image of**)を省略し，単に「これは〜です」(**This is**)としても意味は変わらない．1〜5はいずれも，**an image of**を削除して語数を減らしている．

▌<u>It is said that</u> the temperature will reach 30 degrees.
▌<u>It is thought that</u> the temperature will reach 30 degrees.

1. <u>People think that</u> the temperature <u>will probably reach</u> 30 degrees.
2. <u>We think</u> the temperature <u>will probably</u> reach 30 degrees.
3. The temperature <u>will probably reach 30 degrees</u>.

The expressions **it is said** and **it is thought** are too indirect. They are also unclear because it is not stated who the speaker is. These expressions are commonly found in academic papers and are too formal for oral presentations. Example 3 is the shortest. **The temperature will probably reach 30 degrees**.

「〜といわれている」「〜と考えられている」(**It is said / It is thought**)は論文では多用されるが，口頭発表で用いるには堅苦しい表現である．また，間接的で，発言者が不明確な表現でもある．口頭発表では，発言者を明確にした能動態の文に変更するか（**1**, **2**），この部分を省略してより単純な文にする（**3**）とよい．

How to reduce the level of formality in your presentation
書き言葉の英語を話し言葉の英語に変換する方法

■ Machine accuracy is represented by this equation.

1. This equation represents machine accuracy.
2. Here we have machine accuracy. (Use the pointer to highlight the equation)

In this case, the presenter uses the pointer to indicate the equation and uses the simple sentence Here we have machine accuracy. The expression Here we have is extremely useful for describing what is on a powerpoint slide.

元の文章は受動態であるが、1は語順を入れ替えて能動態の文にしている。

スライド内の数式が何を表しているかを最も簡単に説明するには、2のように、数式をレーザーポインターで指しながら「これは〜です」(Here we have) と言えばよい。

■ We could demonstrate an increase in efficiency of over 12 percent.

1. There was an increase in efficiency of over 12 percent.
2. There was a 12 percent increase in efficiency.
3. Efficiency increased by over 12 percent.

The expression we could demonstrate has been deleted. The word could is redundant. Example 1 is much simpler and starts with There was. The shortest sentence is Efficiency increased by over 12 percent.

1〜3とも、「〜を示すことができた」(We could demonstrate) の部分を省略して語数を減らしている。

■ More powerful batteries are required.

1. We need more powerful batteries.

The sentence has been changed from passive to active. The verb required has been changed to need.

「〜が求められる」「〜が必要とされる」は、受動態の are required ではなく、能動態の We need で表現する。

■ Stable cells <u>are required for</u> IPS regulation.
■ IPS regulation <u>requires</u> stable cells.

1. <u>**For IPS regulation, you need**</u> stable cells.
2. <u>**You need**</u> stable cells for IPS regulation.
3. Stable cells <u>**are necessary for**</u> IPS regulation.

The sentence structure has been changed. The verb **required** has been changed to **need**.

前の例と同様に，required の代わりに need や necessary を用いている．

■ A landslide occurred.

1. <u>**There was**</u> a landslide.

Example 1 starts with **there was**, and the word **occurred** has been deleted.

「地滑りが起こった」(A landslide occurred) を「地滑りがあった」(There was a landslide) と言い換えることで，occurred を削除している．

■ With this system, <u>it is possible to achieve a high degree of accuracy</u>.

1. <u>**This system is highly accurate**</u>.
2. <u>**Using this system, you get a high degree of accuracy**</u>.
3. <u>**There is a high degree of accuracy with this system**</u>.

The phrase **It is possible to achieve** has been deleted. Example 1 is the shortest sentence and the easiest to say.

It is possible to achieve は冗長で堅苦しい表現なので，1～3 はいずれも他の表現に置き換えている．

■ The rocket <u>receives</u> 5 forces.

1. <u>There are 5 forces on the rocket</u>.

文の構造を変え，**There are** で始まる文にしている．

The structure of the sentence has been simplified using the pattern **There are**. The word **receives** has been deleted.

■ A new approach was developed <u>that achieved</u> improved values.
■ A new method was developed <u>that realized</u> improved values.

1. <u>Using this new method</u>, <u>we got</u> improved values.
2. <u>Using this new method</u>, <u>we obtained</u> improved values.

受動態から能動態に変換し，動詞も **achieved**, **realized** から **got**, **obtained** に変えている．**got**（**get** の過去形）は口語的な表現で，口頭発表では多用される．

The words **developed**, **achieved** and **realized** have been deleted. Example 1 is easier to say. The verbs **got** and **obtained** have been used in an active sentence using **we**. The word **got** is informal and frequently used.

■ Biodegradable samples were successfully produced.

1. <u>We produced</u> biodegradable samples.
2. <u>We were able to produce</u> biodegradable samples.

1, 2 とも **We** で始まる能動態の文に変換している，**successfully**（うまく，首尾よく）のニュアンスを残したい場合は，2 のように **We were able to produce** とするとよい．

The sentence has been changed from passive to active using **we**. The word **successfully** has been deleted. In example 2, the phrase **we were able to produce** covers the meaning of the word **successfully**.

Part 3
Simple ways to improve your slides
スライド改善のポイント

In this section, I introduce ways of improving your slides.

　スライドを作成する際，文法や英語表現に関するいくつかの簡単なルールを守ることで，より適切なスライドを作り上げることができます．本章では，スライド作成の際に注意したい 11 のポイントを紹介します．

1 Number your slides
スライドに番号をつけよう

Numbering your slides makes it is <u>**easier for the audience to ask questions**</u>. You can do it like this **1/12**, or like this **1**. The top right-hand side of the slide is a common position. The bottom right is also possible. Here are some examples of questions where a slide number is referred to in the Q and A session.

（聴衆からの質問）　○番目のスライドについて質問があります.

> Step 1　　　　　　　　　　Step 2
>
> ■ <u>I have a question about slide 7</u>. What is the average increase in temperature?
> ■ <u>My question is about slide 7</u>. What is the average increase in temperature?
> ■ <u>Could you show me slide 7, (please)?</u>　What is the meaning of the data in column 2?
> ■ <u>In slide 7, you showed us some data on reliability.</u>　Does that include all experiments?

In the above examples, **there are 2 steps**. In step 1, **the speaker refers to the slide number**. In step 2, **the speaker asks a short, direct question**. This 2-step system makes it easier for people to ask questions, and reduces the chances of miscommunication.

> **Note**　It is **not correct to say** *page* 7. The correct expression is **slide 7**.
> Also please note that the pattern, <u>**Could you show me slide 7?**</u>, is more frequent than the pattern, <u>**Please show me slide 7**</u>. Both are grammatically correct. There is no difference in meaning.

スライドに番号をつけることで，聴衆がスライド番号を指定して質問することができるため，質疑応答を効率的に行える.

2 A space is needed between a number and a word

数字・記号と単語の間にはスペースが必要

If you use a number and a word in the slide title, you should avoid the following mistake.

> スペースなし
>
> ✕ 2.Research goals
> ○ 2. Research goals
>
> スペースあり

There is no space between the period and the following word. This is a relatively minor error but it looks bad. Here is another example.

> スペースなし
>
> ✕ Travel record: time, position(longitude).
> ○ Travel record: time, position (longitude).
>
> スペースあり

You will note that there is no space between the word **position** and the **parenthesis**.

数字と単語の間，記号（ピリオドや括弧など）と単語の間には，必ずスペースを入れる.

3 Use the slide title box to show the section

スライドの最上部のスペースを
上手に活用しよう

At the top of a slide, there is a box for the title. Recently, I noticed that presenters make use of the **top left part of the slide to indicate the part of the presentation** such as **Introduction**, **Results 1**, **Results 2**, **Discussion**. This will help your audience to follow the structure of the presentation. Here are some examples.

- **Introduction**: Research background
- **Results 1**: Data on erosion / Erosion data
- **Results 2**: Data from field studies / Field study data
- **Discussion**: The issue of diffusion / Diffusion

Using the title box to indicate the part of the presentation is a useful technique that helps the audience to follow.

スライドの最上部のスペースには，Introduction，Methods，Results など，そのスライドの内容を記載することで，聴衆が発表の構成を把握しやすくなる．

Use of the definite article the in slide titles
スライドタイトル中の定冠詞 the の使い方に注意しよう

I am often asked about the use of definite articles. It is difficult to give rules that work for every situation, but I would like to point out one issue that concerns the use of articles in slide titles.

> **Example slide titles**
> ▍ The modified apparatus
> ▍ The advantages of the system
> ▍ The measurement procedure
> ▍ The open-case method

In the above examples, the sentences start with the definite article **the**. Titles in powerpoint presentations are generally <u>as short as possible</u>, and <u>definite articles are often omitted to reduce the length</u> of the sentence. So, **The modified apparatus** should be **Modified apparatus**. However, when you are introducing the slide, <u>you use</u> the definite article **the**. Let's look at an example of a <u>slide title and a script</u>.

> **Slide title** Modified apparatus
> **Script** So, let's move on to the next slide. <u>Here we have the modified apparatus</u>. As you can see, it consists of 6 items and the overall size has been reduced by about one third.

In the script, the definite article **the** is used before 'modified apparatus', but in the slide it is omitted.

スライドタイトルは，できる限りシンプルな表現にするために，定冠詞 the は省くことが多い．その場合も，口頭で読み上げる原稿には the を入れるようにする．

5 Using contractions on slides: These samples aren't biodegradable

スライドでは短縮形を使わないようにしよう

Contractions are sometimes called **short forms**. They are used in everyday conversation and informal writing such as text messages. They are generally not used in formal writing, such as academic papers, poster presentations, and powerpoint slides. Here are some examples.

> 短縮形
>
> ✕ We couldn't get a clear image of the reaction.
> ○ We could not get a clear image of the reaction.
>
> 非短縮形
>
> ✕ It's important to weigh the sample first.
> ○ It is important to weigh the sample first.
>
> ✕ This setup doesn't have a temperature gauge.
> ○ This setup does not have a temperature gauge.

This means that **you should not use a short form** in your powerpoint slides. However, it is common to use short forms when you are speaking.

It is → It's などの短縮形は口語的な表現なので，学会発表のスライドには使用できない．ただし，スライドを口頭で説明する際は使用しても問題ない．

Slide title: Singular or plural? 's' or no 's'?

6

スライドタイトルは単数形？ それとも複数形？

Incorrect use of singular and plural nouns is common in slide titles. When introducing a topic <u>for the first time</u>, it is normal to use <u>plural</u> nouns because a general statement is being made. In the following 3 examples, the nouns **measurement**, **battery** and **neuron** should be plural. As this information is being introduced for the first time, <u>the plural noun is used as a general statement</u>. The singular noun is used in a case that is specific.

単数形

× The importance of reliable measurement
○ <u>**The importance of reliable measurements**</u>

複数形

× How to evaluate lithium battery
○ <u>**How to evaluate lithium batteries**</u>

× What is neuron?
○ <u>**What are neurons?**</u>

× Advantage of the revised system
○ <u>**Advantages of the revised system**</u>

名詞の単数形と複数形の使い分けには注意を要する．その単語が指すもの全体についての一般的な話をする場合は複数形を，ある特定のもののみについての話をする場合は単数形を用いる．

7 The word of can be a problem
前置詞 of の使い方に注意しよう

The word **of** is frequently misused in slide titles. Here are some examples.

> この of は誤り

✕ Concept *of* study
○ **Study concept/concepts**

> 語順を入れ替え，of を削除する

✕ Introduction *of* research
○ **Research introduction**

✕ Background *of* research
○ **Research background**

✕ Experiment *of* wave form
○ **Wave form experiments**

In the following 2 examples, the words __introduction__ and __approaches__ are followed by __to__ and not __of__.

X Introduction *of* carbon nanotubes
O **Introduction to carbon nanotubes**

> introduction の後ろは to が正しい

X Approaches *of* TAG production
O **Approaches to TAG production**
O **TAG production**

The correct preposition after the word **approaches** is **to**. It is possible to delete the word approaches and shorten the title to **TAG production.**

X Increase *of* self-sufficiency
O **Increase in self-sufficiency**

> increase の後ろは in が正しい

X Increase *of* temperature
O **Increase in temperature**
O **Temperature increase**

The word __increase__ takes the preposition __in__. For example, There was __an increase in temperature of__ 2 degrees. There was __an increase in yield of__ 20 percent.

前置詞 of を誤って使用してしまうケースは非常に多い．語順を入れ替えて of を削除したほうがよい場合，of 以外の前置詞を使うのが正しい場合（例：introduction to, approaches to, increase in）などに気をつける．

7 The word of can be a problem 前置詞 of の使い方に注意しよう

8 Avoid using the words my or our in slides
スライドでは my や our を用いるのはやめよう

As a general rule, it is better not to use **my** or **our** in slide titles. Here are some examples.

> スライド内では my は使用しない

✗ My experimental set up
○ Experimental setup

✗ Our current research status
○ Current research status

 Note In the above examples, the words **my** and **our** are unnecessary. For more examples see page 16. Column: The word **my** is frequently misused.

スライド内では通常，my や our は使用しない．詳しくは p. 16 のコラムを参照．

Exclamation marks are not used in academic presentations or written papers
エクスクラメーションマークは学会発表では使用しない

Exclamation marks are used after a sentence, word or expression that expresses, **surprise**, **anger** or **excitement**, and are usually not used in academic English in either papers or presentations. However, I often see examples like these.

> ✗ Yield reached 10 per cent!!!
> ✗ We achieved an increase of 25 degrees!!!
> ✗ Thank you for your attention!!!!!!!

This use of exclamation marks creates an unprofessional, casual impression. In the examples given here, the exclamation marks have no meaning or function, and should be deleted.

エクスクラメーションマーク（感嘆符）はくだけた印象を与えてしまうので，学会発表や論文などの学術的な場では使用しないほうがよい．

10 Problems with question marks: Is this a statement or a question?

クエスチョンマークの誤用に注意しよう

Many presenters use questions in their slides in order to get the attention of the audience. This is good because it focuses the audience's attention on a specific point. Here are some examples of mistakes where question marks are not needed.

> How to ... は疑問形ではないので？は誤り

✗ How to evaluate field measurements?
○ How can we evaluate field measurements?

> この文は疑問形なので？が必要

✗ How to develop a more reliable system?
○ How can we develop a more reliable system?

In both of the above examples, the sentences **are not questions. They are statements.** The pattern **How to + verb** is not a question. To turn these sentences into questions, you need to add the question word **can**.

94　Part 3 ● Simple ways to improve your slides　スライド改善のポイント

Here are some more examples.

✕ How to achieve higher efficiency?
◯ How can higher efficiency be achieved?
◯ How can we get/obtain higher efficiency?

✕ Where to position the detector?
◯ What is the best place to position the detector?

✕ Why a catalyst is important?
◯ Why is a catalyst important?

It is important to check if the sentence you put on a slide is a question or not. I frequently see presenters put a question mark after a sentence that is a statement and not a question.

クエスチョンマークは聴衆の興味を引きつけるのに有用であるが，疑問形ではない文章につけるのは誤りなので注意する．

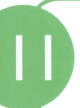

Summary sentences at the bottom of slides: How to reduce the number of words
スライド下部に簡単なまとめを入れよう

It is common to put a summary sentence at the bottom of some slides. However, some presenters use full sentences with difficult vocabulary, which makes it hard for the audience to follow. These sentences sometimes take up a lot of space and make the slides look busy.

Here, I show how to reduce the length of summary sentences. First, **I show the original sentence**, then **the revised sentence** and **the script**.

Example 1

Original sentence ▶ 改善前のまとめ文，このままでは長すぎる
We consider that reliability increases over a wide range.

Revised sentence ▶ 改善後のまとめ文，語数を減らし簡潔にした
Reliability increases over a wide range.

Script ▶ 上記まとめ文を説明する際の原稿例
I'd like to stress that **reliability increases over a wide range.**

In example 1, the expression, **We consider that**, has been deleted from the original sentence. This reduces the length of the sentence.

Example 2

Original sentence

A new system of measurement was developed with improved accuracy of over 15 percent.

Revised sentence

New measurement system improved accuracy by over 15 percent.

Script

So, we developed a new measurement system that improved accuracy by over 15 percent.

In example 2, the original sentence pattern has been <u>changed from passive to active</u>. The word <u>developed</u> has been deleted.

Example 3

Original sentence

It is thought that the addition of an extra catalyst improves the reaction.

Revised sentence

Addition of an extra catalyst improves the reaction.

Script

<u>We found that</u> using an extra catalyst improves the reaction.

In example 3, the expression, <u>It is thought that</u>, has been deleted. This makes the sentence shorter.

11　Summary sentences at the bottom of slides: How to reduce the number of words
スライド下部に簡単なまとめを入れよう

Example 4

> **Original sentence**
>
> **It is suggested that** with early intensive rehabilitation patients can be discharged from hospital up to a week earlier.
>
> **Revised sentence**
>
> Patients having early intensive rehabilitation can leave hospital earlier.
>
> **Script**
>
> With early intensive rehabilitation patients can be discharged a week early.

The expression, **It is suggested**, has been deleted.

The easiest way to reduce the number of words in a summary slide is to delete expressions such as these: **we consider that**, **was developed**, **it is thought that**, **it is suggested that**.

スライドの下部にまとめを 1 文入れることで，聴衆が内容を理解しやすくなる．なるべく簡潔な文になるよう，難しい単語を避け，語数も減らすとよい．

Column #03

A Summary-box and mini-summary can help the audience follow your presentation

Summary-box と mini-summary を活用しよう

It's late October, and I am seeing over 10 presentations a week. Last week's standout presentation was by an associate professor at a national university on the subject of cancer cells. I found the content matter to be quite challenging, but the presenter did two things that really helped me to follow. <u>The first one was to provide summaries at the bottom of some but not all slides.</u> Summary boxes are especially useful at the end of a sequence of slides.

Here is an example.

> **Summary-box の例**
>
> Single infection of vectors make it possible to induce safe differentiated cells efficiently

<u>The use of summary boxes helped me to understand the presentation.</u>

Another technique that I found really useful was <u>the presenter's use of mini-summaries.</u> Typically, the presenter provided short mini-summaries of important information <u>at the end of a section including several slides.</u> <u>Here are some example sentences used by the presenter to signal the start of a mini-summary.</u>

> **Mini-summary を述べる際の表現の例**
>
> ▌ <u>Taken together this data shows the following:</u> + (list of main points)
> ▌ <u>I' ll summarize the significance of these results.</u> + (list of main points)
> ▌ <u>In total this means that...</u>
> ▌ <u>Taken as a whole this means that...</u>
> ▌ <u>Totally, this information suggests that...</u>

発表中に適宜まとめを挟むことで，聴衆が内容を理解しやすくなる．次の２つの
テクニックを上手に活用しよう．

> Summary-box：スライド下部にテキストボックスを設け，簡単なまとめを入れる．全て
> のスライドに加える必要はなく，１つ１つの話題が終わるタイミングで挿入するとよい．
> Mini-summary：口頭で簡単なまとめを述べる．こちらも１つ１つの話題が終わるタイミ
> ングで挟むと効果的である．

Part 4

How to improve the clarity of the main body

本論を分かりやすく伝える方法

The main body is the longest part of an oral presentation. It contains a lot of information and, unless it is carefully structured, can be difficult for the audience to follow. The examples in this section will **improve the clarity of the main body**.

発表の本論（main body）にはたくさんの情報が含まれるため，それらを的確に整理し，聴衆に分かりやすく伝えることが求められます．この章では，論理展開を示す表現，スライド内の情報を説明する表現など，本論の説明に必要な表現と例文を紹介します．

Starting a new topic, section
新しい話題／セクションを始める

The sentences introduced in this section are important because they help the audience to understand the structure of the presentation.

本項では話題の転換に用いる表現を紹介する．これらの表現を活用することで，聴衆が発表の構成を把握しやすくなる．

How to introduce a new section / topic
新しい話題／セクションに移る

続いて，〜についてお話しします．

So that's all I have to say about the methods we used.
- Next, I'm going to **move on to** the results and discussion.

Examples
- Now, I'm going to **go on to** the results and discussion.
- Next, I'm going to **look at** the results and discussion.
- Next, I want to **look at** the results and discussion.
- **Let's look at** the results and discussion.
- **Let's take a look at** the results and discussion.

次の話題／セクションに移る際は，（句動詞）＋（話題／セクション）の形で述べるとよい．句動詞は move on to, go on to, look at, take a look at を用いるのが一般的である．話題／セクションの部分は，the next section（次のセクション）とするか，part 3 や the results and discussion のように具体的な番号／内容を示す．

The most common verbs to indicate you are moving on to a new topic or section are as follows: **move on to**, **go on to**, **look at**, **take a look at**. They are usually followed by these expressions: **the next section**, **part 3**, **the results and discussion**, **applications**, **results from experiment 1**.

1.2 How to move on to the next slide
次のスライドに移る

Here, I show how to make a transition to the next slide.

〜については次のスライドでご説明します．

One of our main objectives was to reduce the thickness of the substrate. This required various approaches.
- **We/you can see that information in the next slide**.
- **I'll show you that information in the next slide**.

Examples
- **I'll show you** some **more data on** that **in the next slide**.
- **I'll show you** more **data on** reliability **in the next slide**.
- **I'll show you** some more **reliability data in the next slide**.
- **I'll show you** the approaches we used **in the next slide**.
- **I'll focus on** that data **in the next slide**.
- **I'll introduce** that data **in the next slide**.
- **I'll describe** the reaction **in the next slide**.

「○○については次のスライドでご説明します」は We (You) can see / I'll show you (+ topic) in the next slide で表現する．

 Note　The preposition **on** is used in the following way.

- I'll show you more **data on reliability**.
- I'll give you some **more information on rates of recurrence**.

「〜についての情報／データ」と言いたいときは，前置詞 on を使い左記のように表す．

1　Starting a new topic, section　新しい話題／セクションを始める

Common errors——よくある間違い

✕ *From now on,* I am going to move on to the results and discussion.

✕ *From now,* I am going to move on to the results and discussion.

◯ <u>Next,</u> I am going to move on to the results and discussion.

◯ <u>Now,</u> I am going to move on to the results and discussion.

✕ I'm going to *move to* the results and discussion.

◯ I'm going to <u>move on to</u> the results and discussion.

✕ I'm going to *go to* the results and discussion

◯ I'm going to <u>go on to</u> the results and discussion.

「今から」を *From now on* や *From now* で表すのは学会発表では不自然である. **Next** や **Now** とするのが正しい.

Move to や *go to* は物理的に移動する際に用いられる表現である.「次の話題に移る」と言うときは move on to や go on to で表し, on を省略することはできない.

The expressions *From now on* / *From now* are unnatural in the context of a presentation. It is more natural to use **next** / **now** / **I'm going to move on to**. Please note that *move to* should be **move <u>on</u> to** and that *go to* should be **go <u>on</u> to**. Both <u>move on to</u> and <u>go on to</u> are 3-word verbs and the words **on** and **to** should not be omitted.

1.3 How to introduce a topic that covers several slides: using the expression in the next few slides
複数枚のスライドにわたる話題に移る

In the above section, I focused on **introducing single slides**. In some cases, it will take **several slides** to cover a single topic. You can use the expression, **in the next few slides**, to introduce a topic that covers several slides. This expression tells the audience that you will introduce several slides that cover the same information/topic. **In the next few slides** can be used at the start or end of a sentence. A similar expression is **over the next few slides**. You can be more specific with the expressions: **over the next three slides** and **in the next three slides**. Here is an example.

1つの話題（例：実験Ａの結果）が複数のスライドにわたることもある。その場合、そのことを聴衆に示すため、下記の例文のように言うとよい。

「次の数枚のスライド」は、in the next few slides または over the next few slides で表す。In the next three slides のように、few の代わりに具体的な数字（スライドの枚数）を入れてもよい。いずれの場合も、slides は複数形とすることに注意する。

> 次の数枚のスライドでは、〜についてご説明します。
>
> That covers the main issues of cost and manufacturing.
> - **In the next few slides, I want to focus on** reliability.
>
> **Examples**
> - **In the next few slides, I'll show you** some data on reliability.
> - **In the next few slides, I'll focus on** reliability.
> - **In the next three slides, I'll talk about / discuss** the issue of reliability.
> - **I'll show you** some data on reliability **in the next few slides**.
> - **Over the next few slides, I'll focus on** reliability.
> - **In the next few slides, I'll discuss** modifications to the system.

1 Starting a new topic, section　新しい話題／セクションを始める

2 Explaining what is on a slide
スライド内の情報を説明する

Here I introduce useful expressions for explaining what is on a slide.

2.1 Use the expression Here we have to introduce the main information on a slide
スライド内の情報を説明する

One of the easiest and quickest ways to introduce the main information on a slide is with the expression **Here we have + (information)**. This is an example.

> スライド内の情報を説明する最も簡単な方法は，説明したいものをレーザーポインターで指しながら **Here we have + (information)** と言うことである.

▌ Script（スライド内のデータをレーザーポインターで指しながら説明する例）

This slide shows data taken from our field experiments. Here we have temperature, (here) precipitation and (here) windspeed.

In this example, **here** can be said once only, or repeated three times. Both are possible. In the example below, the word **here** is said only once and not repeated. This makes the sentence shorter. It is important to use the pointer as you speak to indicate temperature, precipitation and windspeed on the slide.

> **Here we have** を使って複数の箇所について1文で連続して説明する際，2回目以降の **here** は省略してもよい.

▌ Script（上記原稿で2回目以降の here を省略した場合）

This slide shows data taken from our field experiments. Here we have temperature, precipitation, and windspeed.

The biggest advantage of the expression **Here we have** is that it avoids the use of difficult expressions such as these:

the bottom right panel shows and the upper left image depicts.
The bottom right panel shows the annual rainfall, can be changed to, Here we have annual rainfall.

Here are 4 examples of formal expressions that can be changed to informal English using the expression, Here we have.

> スライド内の情報を全て口頭で説明する場合，the upper left image (左上の図) のように，スライドのどの部分について話しているかを1つ1つ述べる必要がある．レーザーポインターと Here we have を使って説明することで，この手間を省くことができる．

- The upper left image depicts the annual rainfall. → ■ Here we have annual rainfall.
- The upper line shows the annual rainfall. → ■ Here we have annual rainfall.
- The lower line shows the annual rainfall. → ■ Here we have annual rainfall.

The underlined expressions on the left are too formal, and quite difficult to say. You can avoid them by using the phrase – Here we have annual rainfall. Please remember to use the pointer to show which part of the slide you are referring to.

(レーザーポインターで指しながら) これは〜を示しています．

- Here we have temperature and (here) precipitation.
- Here we have the main results.
- Here are the main results.
- Here we have the experimental setup.
- Here is the experimental setup.

> 1つ目の例文は1文で2つの箇所について説明しているため，2つ目の here は省略しても構わない．

> Here we have の代わりに Here are/is としてもよい．

 Both patterns can be used:
- Here we have the main results.
- Here are the main results.

2 Explaining what is on a slide　スライド内の情報を説明する

A similar sentence to <u>Here we have</u> is <u>This slide shows</u> **+ (topic)**. Some presenters overuse the expression **This slide shows**. You should try to get a balance by using <u>Here we have</u> as well as <u>This slide shows</u>. Please note that <u>This slide shows</u> is usually <u>used once only in each slide to introduce the main topic</u>, which is probably written in the slide box at the top of the slide. It is not appropriate to use it several times in one slide. The expression <u>Here we have</u> can be used **several times in the same slide** to move on to different information. In the example below, **here we have** is used 3 times to focus on different parts of the same slide.

Here we have と似た表現として This slide shows があるが，使い方が異なることに注意が必要である．This slide shows はそのスライド自体のテーマ（例：「実験方法」）を説明する際に用いられるため，通常 1 枚のスライドに 1 回のみ使用される．一方，here we have はスライド内の個々の図表が何を示しているかを述べる際などに用いられ，1 枚のスライドで複数回使用できる．

> ▌ **Script**(同一スライド内で複数回 here we have を使用する例)

<u>Here we have</u> data from the first experiment. <u>And here</u>, (we have) data from the second experiment, which was done ten days later. <u>And over here, we have</u> average values.

Please note that there are 2 ways of saying the second sentence. You can reduce the length of the sentence by saying, <u>And here, data from the second experiment</u>. Or you can say the sentence in full like this. <u>And here, we have data</u> from the second experiment.

Here we have による説明を 2 文続けて行う場合，2 文目は And here, we have 〜 とするが，we have は省略して単に And here, 〜 としても構わない．

> ### Common errors——よくある間違い
>
> ✕ Here *shows* temperature.
> ◯ Here we have temperature.
> ◯ This slide shows temperature.

The word **here** should be followed by **we have**. It is not possible to say *Here shows*.
In the expression **here we have**, the word **we** includes both the presenter and the audience. The expression <u>Here **you** have</u> is possible, but less frequent.

Here shows という言い方は誤り．Here の後には we have が続く（Here you have と言うこともできるが，あまり使われない）．動詞 show は This slide shows の形で用いられる．

2.2 How to move on to other information in the same slide using short questions such as: How about X? What about X?
スライド内の他の項目に話題を移す

Since slides have a lot of information, you need to move logically and clearly through the material shown. Using simple expressions such as **How about X?** and **What about X?** will signal to the audience that you are moving on to another part of the slide. They are particularly useful if you have a lot of information in columns, lists or tables.

> 同一スライド内の他の項目に話題を移す際は，How about X? や What about X? のように疑問形で問いかけるとよい．

Example 1 (話題を移すために疑問文を活用する例1)

In this slide, we have results from four different locations A to D at different times of year. Locations A and B have standard values. <u>How about locations C and D?</u> As you can see, the values for C and D are quite different. For example, windspeed and temperature were significantly higher.

Example 2 (話題を移すために疑問文を活用する例2)

<u>Here we have</u> the main data from groups A and B. The values are what we would expect. <u>In other words</u>, there are no significant changes. <u>How about group C?</u> Well, at this point, we start to see some significant differences. <u>I'll look at</u> those differences in the next slide.

Using the expressions **How about X?** and **What about X?** helps to avoid a flat, monotonous presentation. There is no difference in meaning between the questions **How about X?** and **What about X?**

> 疑問形を活用することで，発表が単調になるのを防ぐことができる．

2.3 How to introduce another topic in the slide using as for, in terms of, in the case of, as far as, from the viewpoint of
スライド内の他の話題に言及する

In this section, the expressions can be used to introduce other information or topics on the same slide.

Script(As forを用いて新しい話題に言及する例)

We have seen that the apparatus is more reliable, and also robust, particularly at low temperatures. As for energy consumption, it is marginally more efficient.

In the above example, a new topic **energy consumption** is introduced with the expression **as for**. Other expressions are listed below.

一方，○○（今まで説明していたのとは別の話題）については，〜です.

- **As for** energy consumption, it is marginally more efficient.
- **In terms of** energy consumption, it is marginally more efficient.
- **As far as** energy consumption **is concerned**, it is marginally more efficient.
- **From the viewpoint of** energy consumption, it is marginally more efficient.
- **From the** energy consumption **point of view**, it is marginally more efficient.
- **Regarding** energy consumption, it is marginally more efficient.
- **Concerning** energy consumption, it is marginally more efficient.
- **In the case of** energy consumption, it is marginally more efficient.

「一方〜については」という形で新しい話題に移るときは，左記のいずれかの表現を用いるとよい. **As for** と **in terms of** が最も簡単であり，使用頻度も高い.

Part 4 ● How to improve the clarity of the main body　本論を分かりやすく伝える方法

Of these expressions, **as for** and **in terms of** are shorter, easier to say, and more frequently used.

> **Note** The expression **in the case of** requires the word **the**. The expression **in case of** is used like this. **In case of fire, leave the building immediately.** You cannot say *In case of energy consumption*. The correct expression is as follows: **In the case of energy consumption.** Correct use of the definite article **the** is important when using the expression **in the case of**.

In the case of とよく似た表現に in case of があるが，in case of は in case of fire（火事の場合）のように「万が一〜が起こった場合は」というニュアンスをもつ．単に「〜の場合は」と言いたいときは in the case of を用いる．

2.4 Explain what is on the slide: Using the expressions X is in blue and X is shown in blue
文字／線の色について説明する

Information shown on a slide is often represented by a **color**, **type of font**, or **type of line** such as a dotted line. Here I focus on easy ways to introduce what is on a slide **when it is represented by a color**, **type of font** or **type of line**.

口頭発表のスライドでは文字色の違いが何らかの意味をもつことが多い（例：数値が増加した箇所を青字で示す）．そのため，文字色の違いが何を示しているのか，左記のような表現を用いて説明する必要がある．

> **変更箇所は青字で表示しています．**
>
> This is the previous experimental setup. On the right we have the updated setup.
> ▮ Modifications to the system **are in** blue.
> ▮ Modifications to the system **are shown in** blue.

As you can see from the example, the expressions **are in + color** and **are shown in + color** are used. The meaning is the same.

文字や線の色について説明したいときは are in（＋色名）または are shown in（＋色名）と言えばよい．

Here are some examples that use more formal verbs: **show**, **indicate**, **depict**, **represent**. These examples are grammatically correct, but are more appropriate for a written paper than an oral presentation.

2 Explaining what is on a slide　スライド内の情報を説明する

- The blue line <u>shows</u> modification to the system.
- The blue line <u>indicates</u> modifications to the system.
- The blue line <u>depicts</u> modifications to the system.
- The blue line <u>represents</u> modifications to the system.

左記のように show, indicate, depict, represent も「青い線は〜を示しています」の形で色の説明に用いることができるが，やや堅苦しい表現であり，口頭発表には不向きである.

Each of the above 4 sentences can be changed to less formal patterns like these. **Modifications to the system are (shown) in blue.**

2.5 Explain what is on the slide: using in italics, in bold, in large font, underlined, by a dotted line
文字のフォント／線の種類について説明する

Here are some examples using the expressions **in italics**, **in bold**, **in large font**, **underlined** and **by a dotted line**. These are useful expressions for focusing on particular information on a slide. The grammar pattern is the same as **are in blue** or **are shown in blue.**

〜は○○（フォント／線の種類）で示しています.

- Values are **in italics** / **are shown in italics**.
- Values are **in bold** / **are shown in bold**.
- Values are **in large font** / **are shown in large font**.
- Values are **underlined**.

フォント（太字，イタリックなど）の説明は，文字色と同じく，are in（＋フォントの種類）や are shown in（＋フォントの種類）と言えばよい.

> (Note) In this example, the word underline is a verb. The following expressions are incorrect:
>
> ✗ *Values are shown in underlined.*
> ✗ *Values are in underlined.*

下線については動詞 underline を用いて are underlined で表す. 色名／フォント名とは異なり, are (shown) in（＋名詞)の形は使えないことに注意する.

▌Values <u>are shown by a dotted line</u>.
▌Values <u>are represented by a dotted line</u>.
▌<u>The dotted line shows</u> values.
▌<u>The dotted line represents</u> values.

線の種類（破線など）を説明する場合は are shown/represented by（＋線の種類）または（線の種類）＋ shows/represents で表す。

> **Note** The sentence, <u>Values are represented by a dotted line</u>, is quite long and not easy to say. You can avoid this and other sentences introduced in this section with the expression, Here we have values. Please remember to use the pointer as you say <u>Here we have values</u>.

あるいは，線をレーザーポインターで指しながら Here we have（これは〜です）と言うことでより簡単に説明することもできる。

2.6 How to refer to circles, triangles, squares, dots and arrows
グラフや図の中の記号を説明する

In graphs and figures, **circles, triangles**, **squares**, **dots** and **arrows** are used to indicate information. Here are some example sentences.

○○（記号の種類）は〜を表しています．

▌The <u>red circles</u> show temperature.
▌The <u>triangles</u> indicate rate of increase.
▌The <u>squares</u> show rate of increase.
▌The <u>dots</u> indicate rate of increase.
▌The <u>arrows</u> show areas of friction.

グラフや図の中の記号（丸，三角，矢印など）が何を示しているかの説明は，左記のように（記号名）＋ show/indicate と言えばよい．

In the above examples, **circles, triangles, squares, dots, and arrows are plural**. When explaining a graph or figure, in most cases you will use the plural form of **nouns** such as **circles, triangles, squares, dots** and **arrows**. This is because figures will normally have more than one circle, triangle, dot, square or arrow. The same is true for figure legends in papers. Of course, if there is only one circle, the correct exam-

通常，1つのグラフ／図の中には複数の記号が存在するため，記号の名称は複数形で表す（例：circles, arrows）。もちろん，図の中に1つしかその記号が存在しない場合には単数形となることに注意する。

2 Explaining what is on a slide　スライド内の情報を説明する　　113

ple is as follows: **The red circle shows temperature**. But the frequency of this example is very low, since the majority of figures will have more than one circle.

> **Common errors──よくある間違い**

✗ The *circle* shows temperature at various time points.
◯ The **circles** show temperature at various time points.

In most figures, you will have <u>**several circles, dots or triangles**</u>. You cannot say, <u>**the circle shows**</u> if there is more than one circle in the figure.

図の中に複数の丸が存在する場合には，左記の **The** *circle* **shows** のように単数形を用いるのは誤りである。

✗ Values are *written* in red.
◯ Values **are in red**.
◯ Values **are shown in red**.

I frequently hear presenters say, *Values are written in red*. This is incorrect. It should be, **Values are in red** or **Values are shown in red**.

スライド内の文字色を説明する際に **are** *written* **in** とするのは誤りである．正しくは **are in** または **are shown in** となる。

How to use the word mean
動詞 mean の正しい使い方

3.1 Mean: Common errors 1
Mean の誤用例（1）：スライド内のオブジェクトの説明

I'll start this section by focusing on common errors. The first involves using **means** to describe what is on a slide.

✗ The X axis *means* temperature.
◯ The X axis <u>shows</u> temperature.
◯ <u>Here we have</u> temperature.

✗ The dotted line *means* values.
◯ The dotted line <u>represents</u> values.
◯ Values <u>are represented by</u> a dotted line.
◯ <u>Here we have</u> values.

✗ This graph *means* the dry weight of the sample.
◯ This graph <u>shows</u> the dry weight of the sample.
◯ <u>Here we have</u> the dry weight of the sample.

✗ The black circles *mean* rates of biodegradability in the samples.
◯ The black cirlces <u>show / indicate / represent / denote</u> rates of biodegradability in the samples.

The above examples show that **mean** cannot be used to describe something physical on a slide such as **the X axis**, **values**, **dry weight of the sample** or **rates of biodegradability**. In that case, you need to use the words **show**, **indicate**, **depict** and **represent**. It is also easier and quicker to use the expression **here we have + <u>temperature</u>, <u>values</u>,**

スライド内の情報を説明する際，動詞 mean（意味する）を誤って使用しているケースは多い．

動詞 mean は，情報やデータの意味を説明する際に用いる．すなわち，「この実験結果は〜ということを意味しています」のような文で使うのが正しい．左記の例のように，「X軸は〜を示しています」「破線は〜を表しています」など，スライド内のオブジェクトが何を示しているかを説明する場合は，*mean* ではなく show，indicate，depict，represent，denote を用いるのが正しい．

スライド内のオブジェクトを説明する場合は，それをレーザーポインターで指しながら **Here we have** と言うのが最も簡単である（pp. 106〜108 参照）．

3 How to use the word mean　動詞 mean の正しい使い方　115

the dry weight of the sample, rates of biodegradability.

3.2 Mean: Common errors 2
Mean の誤用例（2）：略語の説明

Another common error with the word **mean** is as follows. In this case, people use the word **mean** to explain an acronym.

✗ AIST *means* Advanced Institute of Science and Technology.

○ AIST stands for Advanced Institute of Science and Technology.

○ AIST is short for Advanced Institute of Science and Technology.

In this case, means cannot be used to introduce acronyms. The best way to introduce an acronym is with **stand for** or **is short for**.

Acronym（アクロニム）は頭字語のことで，頭文字をつなげてつくられた略語のことである。「AIST とは～という意味です／の略です」のようにアクロニムの正式名称を説明する際には，*mean* ではなく，stand for か is short for を用いる（p. 180 参照）。

3.3 Using mean to signal the start of an explanation
Mean の正しい使い方（1）：説明の導入として疑問文で使う

Please note that **mean can be used in a question to signal the start of an explanation**. In the examples below, the presenter indicates that what follows is an explanation of data or information already presented.

この結果は何を意味しているのでしょうか？

▌ What do the results mean?

▌ What do these figures mean?

▌ What does the sudden increase in temperature mean?

口頭発表では，結果について説明する際，左記のように What do ～ mean? と疑問形の文を用いることで，聴衆の興味を引きつけることができる。

116　Part 4 ● How to improve the clarity of the main body 本論を分かりやすく伝える方法

3.4 Using mean to explain some information or data
Mean の正しい使い方（2）：情報やデータを説明する

Mean is usually used to **explain some information or data**. Here are some examples in context.

Script（提示した情報が何を意味しているのかを説明する例1）

The brown staining shows that the sample has started to degrade. You can see the evidence of extensive brown staining on both sides of the sample. This means that the decomposition process has started.

In this case, the expression **this means that** is used to explain the information/data that has just been presented. So the presenter switches from **describing** information to **explaining that information** using the expression **This means that**.

Here is another example.

Script（提示した情報が何を意味しているのかを説明する例2）

If you look at the surface of the metal you can see some faint lines. Observation with a microscope shows that the lines penetrate toward the center of the sample. This means that the metal is fractured, and the risk of metal fatigue is extremely high.

In this example, the sentence, **Observation with a microscope shows that the lines penetrate toward the center of the sample**, is explained with the expression, **This means that the metal is fractured, and the risk of metal fatigue is extremely high**.

上記の２つの例のように，mean は情報やデータが何を意味しているかを説明する際に用いられる．上記の例はいずれも，「情報の提示」（例：～という観察結果が得られた）→「情報の説明」（例：この結果は～ということを意味している）の順番になっており，mean は後者の文で使用する．

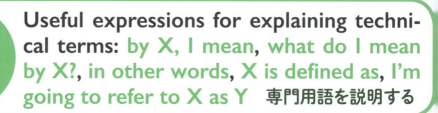

4 Useful expressions for explaining technical terms: by X, I mean, what do I mean by X?, in other words, X is defined as, I'm going to refer to X as Y 専門用語を説明する

4.1 Useful expressions for explaining technical terms
専門用語を説明する際に便利な表現

● **By X, I mean** Xの意味は〜です

It is important to explain any technical terms that the audience might not be familiar with. In the example below, a technical term, **relapse**, is introduced with the phrase, **By relapse, I mean** + explanation.

> By (+専門用語), I mean (+説明) の形で用語の定義／意味を説明する。

Script(By X, I mean の形を使って用語 relapse を説明する例)

> We used different whitening treatments on 3 groups of patients. In groups 1 and 2, teeth remained white after treatment. In group 3, several of the patients suffered relapse. <u>By relapse</u>, <u>I mean</u> the process where the teeth returned to their original color after treatment.

The expression <u>by X, I mean</u> can be used in a question form like this. <u>What do I mean by X?</u> An example of that pattern is shown below.

● **What do I mean by X?** Xはどういう意味でしょうか？

Script(What do I mean by X? の形を使って用語 relapse の説明を始める例)

> <u>What do I mean by relapse?</u> Well, the term relapse refers to a change in the color of the teeth after treatment.

The presenter introduces a technical term with a question **What do I mean by (technical term)?** and then provides a simple explanation of that term.

> 疑問形を使って問いかけてから説明に入ることで、聴衆の興味を引きつけることができる。

Part 4 ● How to improve the clarity of the main body 本論を分かりやすく伝える方法

● In other words　言い換えると／つまり

A less formal way of introducing a technical term is with the expression **in other words**.

> In other words（言い換えると／つまり）を使って用語を説明する.

Script（in other words を使って用語 relapse を説明する例）

Relapse, in other words, the process where the teeth go back to the original color before treatment, is a serious issue.

In this example, the presenter explains a technical term starting with the expression **in other words**.

● X is defined as ＋（short definition）　X は～と定義される

Script（X is defined as の形で X を説明する例）

Relapse is defined as the process where after treatment, the tooth partially returns to its original color.

The expression, (relapse) **is defined as**, is a formal way of explaining something.

> （専門用語）is defined as（＋説明）は用語の定義を説明する改まった表現である.

● I'm going to refer to X as Y　X を Y とよぶことにする

Script（I'm going to refer to X as Y の形で用語 degradation を説明する例）

You can see from the photos of the samples that there are some changes in color and also that the rough surface areas increased. I'm going to refer to this process as degradation.

In some cases, it is necessary to specify how you will refer to something, such as a process or phenomena.

---

④ Useful expressions for explaining technical terms: by X, I mean, what do I mean by X?, in other words, X is defined as, I'm going to refer to X as Y　専門用語を説明する

本日の発表では，X のことを Y とよびます．

- **I'm going to refer to** this process **as** degradation.
- **In this presentation, I'll use the word** degradation **to refer to** changes in color and surface roughness of the samples.
- **I'm going to use the term** degradation **to refer to** changes in color and surface roughness of the samples.

Refer to X as Y で「X（プロセス／現象の説明）を Y（専門用語）とよぶ／という」の意味となる．

左記の 2，3 番目の例文のように，**use the word/term Y to refer to X** の形で用いられることもある．この場合，Y（専門用語）のほうが先に来ることに注意する．

Common errors──よくある間違い

- ✗ *Hereafter,* color change is referred to as degradation.
- ○ In this presentation, **I will refer to color change as** degradation.
- ○ In this presentation, color change **is referred to as** degradation.
- ○ **From here on** / **From now on**, color change **is referred to as** degradation.

The word **hereafter** is very formal and usually used in contracts or legal documents. It means **from here on**, **from now on**. It is too formal to use in an oral presentation. More appropriate expressions are as follows: **in this presentation**, **from here on**, **from now on**. The shortest way of specifying the use of a term or expression is like this. **I will refer to (color change) as (degradation).**

用語の説明で，論文で「以下，〜とよぶ」とするときは hereafter を用いるが，これは堅苦しい表現であり，口頭発表には不向きである．口頭発表で「ここから先は／この発表では〜とよびます」と言いたいときは，「ここから先は／この発表では」の部分は in this presentation, from here on, from now on とし，「〜とよびます」の部分は I will refer to (+説明) as (+用語) とするとよい．

120　**Part 4** ● How to improve the clarity of the main body　本論を分かりやすく伝える方法

4.2 Defining a term using called, known as, referred to as, defined as
「X は Y とよばれる」の形で定義を説明する

There are several expressions for **defining a term**. Here I introduce four of the most frequent: **called**, **known as**, **referred to as**, **defined as**.

Script（calledを用いて用語 relapse を説明する例）

After bleaching, teeth may become several shades lighter. However, it is possible that teeth will partly return to their original color. This process **is called** relapse.

このプロセスは～とよばれます.

▌ This process **is called** relapse.
▌ This process **is known as** relapse.
▌ This process **is referred to as** relapse.
▌ This process **is defined as** relapse.

> X is called Y, X is known as Y, X is referred to as Y, X is defined as Y はいずれも、「X は Y とよばれる」の形で専門用語の説明をする際に用いられる表現である.

In the example, **This process is called relapse**, the word **as** is not used after called.

Common errors──よくある間違い

✗ This process is called *as* degradation.
○ This process **is called** degradation.
○ This process **is known as** degradation.
○ This process **is referred to as** degradation.
○ This process **is defined as** degradation.

> 上記の表現のうち、X is called Y の場合のみ as は不要であることに注意する.

The word **called** cannot be followed by **as**. The word **as** is used like this in the following expressions: **is known as**, **is referred to as**, **is defined as**, but after the word **call**, **as** is not necessary.

---

4 Useful expressions for explaining technical terms: by X, I mean, what do I mean by X?, in other words, X is defined as, I'm going to refer to X as Y　専門用語を説明する

4.3 How to use the word define
動詞 define の使い方

The word **define** occurs frequently in scientific oral presentations. Here are some examples.

私達は〜を〜と定義しました.

- ▌ <u>We define</u> relapse <u>as</u> the degree to which a tooth has reverted to its original color after treatment.
- ▌ We <u>define</u> expert assessors <u>as</u> people with over 25 years' experience of evaluation.
- ▌ For the purposes of this experiment, <u>we define</u> people with over 25 years' experience of evaluation <u>as</u> expert.
- ▌ Expert assessors <u>are defined as</u> people with over 25 years' experience of evaluation.

動詞 define（定義する）は専門用語の定義を説明する際によく用いられる.

動詞 define は受動態で用いると **X is defined as Y** となり，能動態で用いると **we define X as Y** となる. 口頭発表では能動態のほうが適している.

> **Note** In the passive, the pattern is as follows: **X is defined as Y**. For example, **Color change and surface roughness <u>are defined as</u> degradation**. In an active sentence, the structure is, **we define X as Y**. The active sentence, <u>**We define X as Y**</u> is better for oral presentations. For example, <u>**We define color change and surface roughness as degradation**</u>.

122　Part 4 ● How to improve the clarity of the main body　本論を分かりやすく伝える方法

Simplifying and rephrasing the information you present
情報を単純化して伝える／平易な表現に言い換える

An oral presentation is not the same as an academic paper. Readers of an academic paper are in control of the information in front of them, and can reread sections of the paper to check information. The audience at an oral presentation has no control over the information being presented. For this reason, **simplification of the information presented is necessary to help the audience follow**. In this section, I introduce examples of **how to simplify information**.

論文では読者は文章を何度も読み返すことができるが，口頭発表ではそれができないため，発表者は聴衆に一度の説明で理解してもらわなければならない．そのため，必要に応じて情報を平易化・単純化して伝えることが求められる．

5.1 Simplify information using it's a kind of, it's a type of
情報を単純化して伝える

The phrases **It's a kind of**, **It's a type of**, can be used to simplify the material you are presenting. The word **basically** can be added to these expressions like this. **Basically, it's a kind of**, **Basically, it's a type of**. The word **basically** is used to indicate that what follows is a simplification.

学会発表では時間の都合上，論文とは違って全ての内容について厳密で詳細な説明をすることはできない．細かい解説が不要な内容については，単純化して分かりやすく伝えるようにする．その際，It's a kind of / It's a type of（ある種の〜／〜のような），basically（簡単に言うと〜／基本的には〜）を使うことで，情報が単純化・簡略化されたものであることを示すことができる．

Script（使用材料について単純化した説明を行う例）

To measure levels of pollution, we launched balloons with sensors at a height of 100 meters. These were attached to stakes in the ground with the white material seen in the photograph. <u>Basically</u>, the material is made of nylon. <u>It's a kind of</u> fishing line that was developed specifically for this purpose.

In the above example, using the words **basically** and **it's a kind of**, the presenter avoids a detailed explanation of the material used in the experiments to <u>**save time**</u> and <u>**simplify the explanation**</u>.

上記の例では，使用した材料に関する詳細な説明は省き，basically と it's a kind of を用いた簡単な説明で済ませている．こうすることで，説明に要する時間を短縮することができ，また聴衆も理解しやすくなる．

簡単に言うと，〜です．

▮ <u>**Basically, the material is made of**</u> nylon.

▮ <u>**It's a kind of**</u> fishing line.

▮ <u>**It's a type of**</u> fishing line made of nylon.

▮ <u>**Basically, it's a kind of**</u> fishing line made of nylon.

▮ <u>**I won't go into details**</u>. <u>**Basically, it's a kind of / type of**</u> fishing line made of nylon.

In the last example, the expression <u>**I won't go into details**</u> signals a simplification.

最後の例文は I won't go into details（won't は will not の短縮形）の１文を入れることで，詳細には触れず簡単な説明で済ませることを示している．

5.2 Simplifying the material presented with in other words
言い換える／要約する

The expression **in other words** is a useful way of simplifying or summarizing a detailed explanation or a technical term.

Script（言い換えを行っている例）

Notice what happens with the adipic acid. The first proton is more like the proton in acetic acid. <u>In other words</u>, the P-K-A has gone up relative to the P-K-A of succinic acid.

To make your presentation as clear as possible, it is necessary to simplify the material presented. This not only saves time, but also makes it easier for the audience to follow. The most frequently used expression is **in other words**. A similar expression is **to put it simply**. The word **basically** can also be used.

In other words は「言い換えると」「要するに」という意味で，より分かりやすい表現で言い換えるときに用いられる．同様の目的で to put it simply や basically を用いることもできる．

言い換えると／要するに，～です．

▌ <u>In other words</u>, the results we got seem to have a high degree of reliability.

▌ <u>In other words</u>, there is a lot of essential bacteria that is required if we want to degrade plastic in soil.

▌ <u>To put it simply</u>, online questionnaires are a simple way of collecting feedback.

▌ <u>Basically</u>, online questionnaires are a simple way of collecting feedback.

Common errors──よくある間違い

✕ In other *word*, it has a high degree of reliability.
○ In other **words**, it has a high degree of reliability.

The phrase **in other words** is always in the plural. This means you cannot say *in other word* with no **s**.

In other words と言うとき，words は常に複数形で用いることに注意する．*In other word* は誤り．

5 Simplifying and rephrasing the information you present
情報を単純化して伝える／平易な表現に言い換える

125

5.3 How to rephrase your explanation with What I mean is, What I want to say is, So, I mean that, My point is that, I'll just rephrase that　平易な言葉で言い換える

The word **rephrase** means to **say something in different words so that it is clearer**. Rephrasing what you have said will help the audience to follow the points you are making.

動詞 rephrase は「言い換える」という意味で，要点をより平易な表現で言い換える際に用いられる．

言い換えると／つまり，ポイントは〜ということです．

▌ <u>What I mean is that</u> by using this material, battery performance improves.

▌ <u>What I want to say is that</u> by using this material, battery performance improves.

▌ <u>So, I mean that</u> by using this material, battery performance improves.

▌ <u>My point is that</u> by using this material, battery performance improves.

▌ <u>I'll just rephrase that.</u> Using this material, battery performance improves.

言い換えによって要点を強調したい場合は，左記のような表現を用いるとよい．

左記の表現は，発表の途中だけではなく，質疑応答時に発表内容を振り返る場合にも使うことができる．その場合，左記の表現を過去形にする必要があることに注意する．例：What I meant was, What I wanted to say was, My point was that, The point I was making was. 動詞 rephrase を使う場合は，I would like to rephrase what I said about (topic) とするとよい．

In the last example, **rephrase** is a verb.

> **Note** In some cases, such as the question and answer session, you may need to return to something you said and rephrase it. You can use the expressions presented in section 5.3. However, the sentences <u>should be in the past tense</u>. Here are some examples.

▌ <u>What I meant was</u>
▌ <u>What I wanted to say was</u>
▌ <u>My point was that</u>
▌ <u>The point I was making was</u>

+ a short explanation.

If you use the word <u>rephrase</u> as a verb, here is an useful example.

▌ <u>I would like to rephrase what I said about (topic).</u>

126　**Part 4** ● How to improve the clarity of the main body　本論を分かりやすく伝える方法

Giving an estimate using the words about, approximately, in the region of, typical, typically, basically
詳細には触れず，おおまかな数値／一般論を述べる

In this section, I introduce useful words and expressions for giving an estimate and simplifying your explanation.

 About, approximately, in the region of
おおまかな数値を述べる

In some cases, you will not be able to give a precise number or value, because you do not have the data, or because you want to save time and avoid a detailed explanation. Giving an estimate is not a problem as long as you make it clear that the figure is only an estimate. You can use these expressions to **indicate that the information is an estimate**.

- **About**　およそ，約
  - Reported values are <u>about</u> 10 percent.

- **Approximately**　およそ，約
  - Reported values are <u>approximately</u> 10 percent.
  - The reduction in time is <u>approximately</u> 15 minutes.

- **In the region of**　およそ，約，〜の辺り
  - The yearly yield is <u>in the region of</u> one million tons.
  - The reaction time is <u>in the region of</u> 4 to 5 minutes.
  - Reported values are <u>in the region of</u> 10 percent.

口頭発表において数値を述べる際，正確なデータがない場合や細かい数値を読み上げる時間がない場合には，正確な数値ではなくおおまかな数値を述べることになる．その場合，その数値が概算値であることを明確に示す必要がある．

数値が概算値であることを示すためには，左記のいずれかを数値の前につけて表現する．

6.2 How to use the words typical and typically to make a general statement that will simplify your explanation
一般的な数値を述べる

Use the words **typical** or **typically** to give the audience a rough idea of **a number**, **amount**, **quantity**, or **time**. These words are useful because you can avoid detailed explanations by focusing on the main points, or giving an estimate. They are also an easy way of **giving a short answer** in the question and answer session.

> 下記の例のように, ある数量が条件の違いによってさまざまな値をとりうる場合には, 詳細な説明は省き, 最も一般的な値のみを紹介することがある. その際は, そのことを示すために typical や typically を用いる. この方法は質疑応答の際にも有用である.

● Typical 一般的な／典型的な（形容詞）

Script（さまざま数値をとりうることを説明したうえで, 一般的な数値を述べる例）

> The yield from this experiment depends on the location and a few other variables. A typical yield is from 5 to 10 percent.

一般的には／通常は○○（数値など）です.

Examples

▌ **A typical yield is** 5 to 10 percent.
▌ **A typical duration would be** 24 hours.

The word **typical** is usually followed by a noun such as **yield** or **duration**. For example, <u>a typical yield is 10 per cent</u>, <u>a typical duration is 24 hours</u>, <u>a typical increase is 10 grams</u>.

> Typical は形容詞であり, その後ろには数量を表す名詞［例：yield（収率）, duration（継続時間）, increase（増加量）］が続く.

There are two grammar patterns.
1. <u>A typical yield is</u>
2. <u>A typical yield would be</u>
The most frequent pattern is <u>a typical yield is</u>. There is no difference in meaning between these expressions, but the

> A typical 〜 is も A typical 〜 would be も意味はほとんど同じであるが, A typical 〜 is のほうがやや直接的な表現である.

expression **A typical yield would be** is slightly less direct than **A typical yield is**.

Useful expressions are:

▌**A typical yield** is <u>in the region of</u> 10 to 20 percent.
  <u>approximately</u>
  <u>about</u>
  <u>around</u>

▌**A typical yield**   is 100,000 tons.
  <u>duration</u>   is 10 minutes.
  <u>increase</u>   is 15 percent.
  <u>distance</u>   is several kilometres.
  <u>weight</u>   is 15 kilos.
  <u>temperature</u> is 25 degrees.

● Typically   一般的に／典型的に／通常は（副詞）

The word **typically** is frequently used at the beginning of a sentence, but can also be used after a verb. Please note that **typically** is often used in the question and answer session when presenters want to give a **quick, short answer** that involves numbers, time, amount, duration or quantity.

Typically は副詞であり，通常は文頭で用いられるが，動詞（be 動詞を含む）の後ろで用いられることもある.

Typically は質疑応答の際，数値に関する質問に対して簡単に答えたい場合に使われることが多い.

通常は／一般的には○○（数値など）です．

▌<u>Typically,</u> cell culture time is 2 to 3 days.
▌Cell culture time is <u>typically</u> 2 to 3 days.
▌<u>Typically,</u> values are in the region of 5 to 10 percent.
▌Values are <u>typically</u> in the region of 5 to 10 percent.

6 **Giving an estimate using the words** about, approximately, in the region of, typical, typically, basically 詳細には触れず，おおまかな数値／一般論を述べる

6.3 How to use the word basically to simplify your explanation
複雑な内容を単純化して説明する

The word **basically** is used for simplification, and makes it possible to avoid long and complicated explanations. It is also useful for handling difficult questions. Please note that basically is used in **oral and poster presentations**, but **not in academic papers**. Here are some examples.

Script（複雑なプロセスを単純化して簡単に説明している例）

This process is quite complicated. <u>Basically</u>, the materials are stacked on top of each other with adhesive added at each level for stability. <u>This means</u> that stability increases by over 10 percent.

Here, the presenter avoids a detailed description of a complicated process. The word **basically** is used to **introduce a simplified explanation that is short and avoids unnecessary explanation**. In this example, the expression <u>this means</u> signals the start of a brief explanation.

簡単に言うと／基本的に，〜です．

▎ <u>Basically</u>, this system can be used in any situation.
▎ <u>Basically</u>, we take a number of cells, immerse them in solution for 24 hours and measure their activity levels.

In example 2, the presenter uses the word **basically** to indicate that the following short explanation is a simplification of a complicated process.

口頭発表や質疑応答では，複雑な内容をそのまま説明している時間はないことが多い．その場合，内容を単純化／簡略化したうえで，文頭に basically（簡単に言うと／基本的には〜）をつけてそのことを示すとよい．

Basically を使えるのは口頭発表やポスター発表だけで，論文では使用できないことに注意する．

2番目の例文は，basically を文頭に置くことによって，その後に続く実験手順の説明が単純化されたものであること（実際にはもっと複雑であること）を示している．

130   Part 4 ● How to improve the clarity of the main body 本論を分かりやすく伝える方法

7 Skipping information and focusing on the main points
要点の説明に絞り，一部の説明を省略する

If your slides have a lot of detailed information, you may need to skip some of it to save time and simplify your explanation.

7.1 When you need to skip some of the material on a slide
スライド内の一部の情報の説明を省略する

このデータについては説明を省略します.

▌ I'll skip this data.

詳細については省略します.

▌ This slide contains a lot of facts / figures / information / data / material. I'll skip the detail / details.

▌ There is a lot information here. I'll skip the detail / details.

▌ There is a lot of information here. I won't / will not go into detail / details.

スライド内の一部のデータ／図表の説明を省略したい場合は，左記のように言えばよい.

Please note that both **detail** and **details** can be used. Also note the useful expression **to go into detail / details**. In the expression, **I'll skip the details**, the definite article is necessary. The expression, **I will not go into details**, has a two-word verb **go into**.

「詳細は省略する」と言うとき，「詳細」は単数形の detail でも複数形の details でもどちら でもよい. 句動詞 go into を使って I will not / won't go into details と言うときは the は不要であるが，I'll skip the details と言うときは the が必要であることに注意する.

7.2 When you need to skip a slide completely
スライドを飛ばす

時間がないので，このスライドは飛ばします．

- I'll skip this slide.
- I'm running out of time, so I'll skip this slide.
- I only have a few minutes left, so I'll skip this slide.
- Time is limited. So, I'm afraid I'll have to skip the next few slides.

> スライドを丸ごと飛ばすときは左記のように言えばよい．スライド1枚を飛ばすときは1～3番目の例文のように，スライド複数枚を飛ばすときは4番目の例文のように言う．

7.3 When you need to skip details but want to focus on a few main points
詳細の説明は省き，要点のみ説明する

When there is a lot of information on your slide, **you should focus on the main points to help the audience follow, and also to save time**. You should remember that **the audience will rapidly scan the information as you speak**. You do not need to explain everything on the slide in detail.

> 口頭発表では，聴衆は発表者が話している間にスライド全体を確認することが可能なため，発表者は必ずしもスライド内の情報全てを口頭で説明する必要はない．要点のみの説明を行う場合は，そのことを示すため次ページのような表現を用いるとよい．

Part 4 ● How to improve the clarity of the main body　本論を分かりやすく伝える方法

Script(データが多いため要点に絞って説明することを述べている例)

This table shows data collected from 7 different experiments. As you can see, the slide has a lot of information. <u>So, I'll skip the details</u> and <u>focus on the main points</u>, which are as follows: (explain the main points briefly).

詳細は省略して，重要なところだけご説明します．

- <u>There is a lot of information here. So, I'll skip the details and look at</u> the main points, which are as follows: (explain the main points).
- <u>I'll skip the details and (just) mention</u> the important information / the key data.
- Here we have data from group 2, <u>I won't go into details, but the main point is</u> (explain the main point).

 How to use **as follows** and **the following**

1. <u>I'll skip the details and look at</u> the main points, which are <u>as follows:</u>

In this usage, it is important to have an **s** on the word **follow**. The expression **as follows**, is usually followed by a list. *As follow* is a common error.

2. <u>The following points</u> are important.

In this example, the pattern is **the following points**. There is no **s** on the word **following**. You cannot say, The *followings* are important. This is a common error where presenters confuse the two expressions. **As follows** and **the following**.

1番目の例文のように，「要点は以下のとおりです」と言いたいときは，as follows: (+ 要点のリスト) のように言う．この場合，follow は動詞であり，s をつける必要がある．一方，The following points と言う場合は，following は形容詞であり，followings のように s をつけるのは誤りである．

7.4 How to focus on the main points: Using I'll (just) focus on, I'll go over, I'll look at, I'll run through
要点に絞って説明する

Script(要点のみ説明することを focus on で示している例)

In field experiments, we collected data on windspeed, precipitation and humidity at 16 sites over a period of 12 months. Here is the data. <u>There is a lot of detailed information</u>, <u>so I'll just focus on</u> the main points.

● Focus on

- ■ <u>This slide is a bit busy</u>, <u>so, I'll focus on</u> the main points / the key data.
- ■ <u>This slide is somewhat busy</u>, <u>so, I'll focus on</u> the main points / the important information.
- ■ <u>There is a lot of information</u>, <u>so, I'll focus on</u> the main points / the latest data.
- ■ <u>There's a lot of data here</u>. <u>I'll skip the details and focus on</u> the main points.

● Go over

- ■ <u>As you can see, there is a lot of data</u>, <u>so, I'll go over</u> the main points.
- ■ <u>There is a lot of data here</u>. <u>So, I'll go over</u> the main points.
- ■ <u>This slide is rather busy</u>, <u>so, I'll go over</u> the important information.

● Look at

- ■ <u>There is a lot of information here</u>. <u>I'll look at</u> the most recent results.
- ■ <u>There is a lot of data here</u>. <u>I'll look at</u> the results from experiment 2 only.

「詳細は省略して要点のみ説明します」と言いたいときは，左記のいずれかの句動詞を用いるとよい.

Part 4 ● How to improve the clarity of the main body　本論を分かりやすく伝える方法

● Run through

▎ <u>There is a lot of information here</u>. <u>I'll run through</u> the most important results.

▎ <u>There is a lot of data here</u>. <u>I'll just run through</u> the main points.

When you skip data / information and focus on important points, these verbs are frequently used.

▎ There is a lot of data here.
I'll <u>focus on</u> the main points in this slide.
  <u>go over</u>
  <u>look at</u>
  <u>run through</u>
  <u>concentrate on</u>

Here are some expressions that are frequently used in combination with the above verbs.

▎ I'll (just) go over <u>the main points</u>.
         <u>the most recent data</u>.
         <u>the most important data</u>.
         <u>the most important results</u>.
         <u>the most relevant data</u>.
         <u>the key data</u>.
         <u>the essential information</u>.

本項で紹介した句動詞を使って「要点（のみ）を説明する」と言うとき，句動詞の後ろには，左記のように「要点」や「重要なデータ」を表す語句を続ける．

7 Skipping information and focusing on the main points　要点の説明に絞り，一部の説明を省略する

8

How to help the audience follow your presentation by using forward movement, backward movement, and reminders
次に話す内容を予告する／前に話した内容を振り返る

In this section, I introduce useful sentences that will make it easy for the audience to follow the presentation.

> Forward movement（前方への移動＝次に話す内容の説明）と backward movement（後方への移動＝前に話した内容の振り返り）を活用することで，聴衆が発表の構成をつかみやすくなる.

8.1 Forward movement
次に話す内容を予告する

You can help the audience follow your presentation by signaling **forward movement**. The examples below can be used to tell the audience **what will happen in the next few minutes of the presentation**. This helps people to **understand the structure of your presentation**.
These examples are for **referring to information in the next slide**.

> Forward movement（次に話す内容の説明）には，次のスライドで話す内容を予告する場合と，次のセクションで話す内容を予告する場合がある.

〜については次のスライドでお話しします.

- So, the main issue is reliability. **I'll talk about that in the next slide**.
- So, the main issue is reliability. **I'll focus on that in the next slide**.
- So, the main issue is reliability. **That is what I am going to talk about next**.
- So, the main issue is reliability. **That's my next point**.

These examples are for **introducing information in the next section**.

136 **Part 4** ● How to improve the clarity of the main body 本論を分かりやすく伝える方法

～については次のセクションでお話しします.

- **I'll talk about** the significance of this result **in the next section**.
- **I'll look at** the experimental data **in the results**.
- **I'll come back to** this point **in the discussion**.
- **I'll mention this again** in **the materials and methods section**.
- **I'll return to** this issue **later**.
- **I'll introduce some more data on** this topic **later**.
- **I'll show you that information in a moment**.
- **I'll give you some more information about** this **shortly**.

■ Commonly used verbs when introducing forward movement

- **I'll talk about** this issue in the next section / in the results / in part 2.
  explain
  say something about
  look at
  give you some data on
  give you some examples of
  introduce some more data on
- **I'll show** you that data / information / those results in the discussion.
- **I'll come back to** this issue in the next section.
- **I'll return to** this issue in part 3.

■ Commonly used expressions when introducing forward movement

- **I'll talk about** this issue **in the next slide**.
  in the next few slides.
  in the discussion.
  in a moment.
  in a few minutes.
  shortly.
  in the next section / **in part 2**.
  later.
  at the end of the presentation.

8 How to help the audience follow your presentation by using forward movement, backward movement, and reminders　次に話す内容を予告する／前に話した内容を振り返る

8.2 Backward movement
前に話した内容を振り返る

In backward movement, you **remind the audience of information you have already covered**. This **improves the connectivity of the presentation** and **makes your presentation easier to follow and remember**.

How to briefly return to a point you have already made.

> ### 先ほど〜のところでお話ししたとおり，〜です．
>
> ■ **As I mentioned in the background,** typical lifespans for this product are between 5 to 7 years.
>
> ■ **As I said in the background,** typical lifespans for this product are between 5 to 7 years.
>
> ■ **As I explained in the introduction,** typical lifespans for this product are between 5 to 7 years.
>
> ■ **As I pointed out at the beginning of my talk**, typical lifespans for this product are between 5 to 7 years.
>
> ■ **As I told you in part 1,** typical lifespans for this product are between 5 to 7 years.
>
> ■ **As we saw in the previous slide,** this method also has medical applications.
>
> ■ **As we saw previously,** this method also has medical applications.
>
> ■ **Here is the data we saw in experiment 1**. And this is the new data from our most recent experiment. **As you can see,** there are some significant differences.

In the above example, the sentence, **Here is the data we saw in experiment 1**, is used to refer to previously presented material.

Backward movement（前に話した内容の振り返り）を上手に活用することで，前後の内容のつながりが明確になり，聴衆が内容を理解しやすくなる.

前に話した内容を振り返る際は，左記のように **As I**（＋動詞）**in**（＋セクション），〜 の形を使って，「（セクション）のところでお話ししたとおり，（前に話した内容の要約）です」のように述べるとよい.

最後の例文は，スライドに2つの実験の結果（片方は前に説明したもの，もう片方は新しく提示したもの）を示し，前に説明したほうをレーザーポインターで指しながら「こちらは先ほど説明したものです」と言っている例である.

Verbs for **backward movement** are as follows in order of frequency:

As I <u>mentioned</u>, <u>said</u>, <u>told you</u>, <u>explained</u>, <u>pointed out</u>, <u>As we saw</u>

> (Note) The expression, <u>As we saw</u> is a useful way of referring to something you have already said or shown the audience. It is usually used with these expressions. **As we saw in the introduction, background, materials and methods, last section, in experiment 1.**

前に説明した内容を振り返るとき，動詞は左記のいずれかを用いることが多い．動詞として mentioned や said を使う場合は主語は I となり，saw（see の過去形）を使う場合は主語は we となることに注意する．

Commonly used expressions for <u>backward movement</u> are as follows:

▎As I mentioned <u>in the background,</u>   battery performance improves.
<u>in the introduction,</u>
<u>in the previous section,</u>
<u>in part 1,</u>
<u>previously,</u>
<u>in the last section,</u>
<u>a moment ago,</u>
<u>a few minutes ago,</u>
<u>just now,</u>

いつ説明した内容であるかを示すには，in the background や in part 1 のようにセクション名／セクション番号を述べるか，a few minutes ago（数分前）のように言えばよい．

(8) How to help the audience follow your presentation by using forward movement, backward movement, and reminders　次に話す内容を予告する／前に話した内容を振り返る

How to use the expression **go back to** for backward movement.

> ～のところでお話しした内容をもう一度振り返りたいと思います.
>
> ▌ **I'd like to go back to what I said about** medical applications.
> ▌ **I want to go back to the introduction.**
> ▌ **I'll just go back to the results and mention** applications.
> ▌ **I'm going to go back to the experimental setup** and **remind you of** the major differences between these systems.

左記のように, 句動詞
go back to（戻る）を
使うこともできる.

8.3 How to refer back to information already presented using the word remind
重要事項を再度説明する際の表現：remind と reminder

In order to stress the important information in your presentation, it is necessary to remind people of the main points you have already covered.

▌ Script（重要事項を再度説明することを動詞 remind で示している例）

> Ok, so I'd just like to remind you of the material / data / ground / information we have covered. We modified the system with additional battery power. After further tests, we found that processing speed, reliability and usability went up.

In some cases, presenters will support their explanation with notes on a slide like these.

▌ **system was modified using additional battery power**
▌ **processing speed went up**
▌ **reliability and usability improved**

140　Part 4 ● How to improve the clarity of the main body　本論を分かりやすく伝える方法

重要なポイントをおさらいしたいと思います.

■ **I'd just like to remind you of** the material / data / ground / information we have covered.

● Remind

■ **I'd (just) like to remind you of the main points so far**. (＋ short summary)

■ **I want to remind you of the points I made in the last section**. (＋ short summary)

■ **I'd (just) like to remind you of** the results. (＋ short summary)

■ **This is (just) to remind you of** the main points I made in the last section. (＋ short summary)

■ **I want to remind you of** the key data. (＋ short summary)

● Reminder

■ **This is (just) a quick reminder of the main points so far**. ＋ List of main points.

■ **This is a reminder of the main points**. **We found** that temperature increased, and that the reaction was longer. **We also found that** the flexibility of the samples improved.

重要な内容を再度説明することを示す際に便利な表現として, 動詞 remind (思い出させる) と名詞 reminder (思い出させるもの) がある. Remind は I'd (just) like to remind you of the main points (＋簡単なまとめ) の形で, Reminder は This is (just) a reminder of the main points. We found (＋簡単なまとめ)の形で用いる. まとめを口頭で述べるのと併せて, スライドに箇条書きの要点を表示させるとより効果的である.

Common errors──よくある間違い

✕ As I *said you*, reliability is an issue.
○ **As I said,** reliability is an issue.
○ **As I told you** in the introduction, reliability is an issue.

In backward movement, the word **said** is frequently used. After the word **said**, *you* is not necessary. However, if you use the word **told**, it is necessary to use **you**. For example, **As I told you**, degradation is an issue.

「(先ほど) お話ししたとおり」と言うとき, 動詞として said を用いる場合は you は不要 (As I said you は誤り) であるが, told を用いる場合は you が必要 (As I told you が正しい) である.

✕ As I *talked,* cost is an issue.
◯ As I mentioned / said / explained / told you / pointed out, cost is an issue.
◯ As we saw, cost is an issue.

The verb **talk** cannot be used like this. *As I talked.* However, **talked about** can be used in the following examples, where it is preceded by in the previous/last slide. For example, In the introduction, in the previous/last slide, I talked about cost.
I talked about cost in the introduction, in the previous/last slide.

✕ As I *spoke,* cost is an issue.
◯ As I said, cost is an issue.

In this case, **spoke** cannot be used with the expression As I + verb.
However, **spoke about** can be used in the following pattern. In the introduction, I spoke about applications. In this case, spoke about or talked about can both be used. But the frequency of talked about is much higher than spoke about.

「（先ほど）お話ししたとおり」を As I（＋動詞），〜 の形で表すとき，動詞は said や mentioned を用いるが，*As I talked* とするのは誤りである．I talked about を使うことができるのは，その前に In the introduction や In the previous slide がある場合であることに注意する．

As I talked と同様に *As I spoke* も誤りである．I talked about と同様，In the introduction, I spoke about の形で使うことはできるが，この場合 spoke ではなく talked を使うのが一般的である．

9 Focusing on information on the slide
スライドのどこに注目してほしいかを示す

It is necessary to guide the audience through the information on the slide, focusing on key information using **I'd like to focus on**, **Let's take a look at**, **Let's look at** and **Please look at**.

> スライドには多くの情報が含まれることが多い．その中でどこに注目してほしいのか，どこが特に重要なのかを，聴衆に示す必要がある．

9.1 Draw the attention of the audience to important information
スライド内の注目箇所を示す

Script（スライドの注目箇所を示した後，そこから何が読み取れるかを説明する例）

I'd like to focus on the table on the right. It includes data on precipitation. As you can see, September is the wettest month.

This is a 2-step move. In step 1, the presenter focuses on a particular part of the slide with the sentence, **I'd like to focus on** topic. In part 2, the presenter explains the data with the sentence, **As you can see**, September is the wettest month.

> 上の例では，はじめに表に注目してほしいことを I'd like to focus on で述べたうえで，その表から何が読み取れるかを As you can see で説明している．

～にご注目ください．この図表／データから～であることが分かります．

▌ **I'd like to focus on** the table on the right. <u>As you can see,</u> there is a reduction in weight.

▌ **Let's take a look at** the experimental setup. <u>As you have probably noticed,</u> there is a reduction in size.

▌ **Let's look at** the bar chart. <u>As you have probably seen,</u> rates are fairly consistent.

▌ **Please look at** the precipitation data. <u>As you have probably noted,</u> June has become progressively drier.

注目箇所を示すには，I'd like to focus on の他にも，Let's take a look at や Let's look at，Please look at と言うこともできる．

Common errors──よくある間違い

✕ *Please see this figure*.
◯ **I'd like to focus on** this figure.
◯ **Let's take a look at** this figure.
◯ **Let's look at** this figure.

The expression, **Please see this figure**, is incorrect. It would be possible to say, **Please look at**. The most frequently used expression in this case is, **I'd like to focus on**.

「～をご覧ください」を *Please see* と表すことはできない．Please ～ を使うのであれば Please look at とするのが正しい．この場合，I'd like to focus on を使うのが最も一般的である．

144　**Part 4** ● How to improve the clarity of the main body　本論を分かりやすく伝える方法

9.2 How to use the word if to focus on information on the slide
注目箇所／要点を示すための表現（1）：if

The word **if** is frequently used in oral presentations, particularly when explaining information on a slide. **If** is used to draw the attention of the audience to important information on the slide.

> **If** を文頭に置いて「〜をご覧いただくと」の形で注目箇所を示すことができる.

〜をご覧いただくと，〜であることが分かります.

- ■ **If you look at this red line, you will see that** degradation increases rapidly after day 3.
- ■ **If you look at this data, you will notice that** degradation increases rapidly after day 3.
- ■ **If you look at the results for experiment 3, you will see** a sudden increase in dopamine.
- ■ **If we look at the reaction site, we can see** that changing the catalyst causes a dramatic reaction.

> **If** を使う場合は，左記の例文のように If you/we look at (＋注目箇所), you will see/notice/observe/find (＋そこから読み取れる内容) の形とする.

If is usually positioned at the start of the sentence and is used with the verb **look at**. The pattern is as follows: **If you/ we look at**. The second part of the same sentence starts with **you will see** / **notice** / **observe** / **find**.

Common errors——よくある間違い

- ✕ If we *see* figure 2, the temperature increase is clear.
- 〇 If we <u>look at</u> figure 2, we can see that the temperature increase is clear.

- ✕ If you *see* the samples carefully, you can see small fractures in the surface.
- 〇 If you <u>look at</u> the samples carefully, you can see small fractures in the surface.

> **Please look at** の場合と同様に，**if** を使う場合も動詞は **see** ではなく **look at** とするのが正しい.

The word **if** is usually used with <u>look at</u>. It is not used with *see*.

9 Focusing on information on the slide　スライドのどこに注目してほしいかを示す

9.3 Using the words interestingly and interesting to focus on important information
注目箇所／要点を示すための表現 (2)：interestingly, interesting

A flat presentation is difficult to follow because the presenter does not stress the main points. In other words, there is **no hierarchy of main points** and the presentation is **monotonous**. The words **interestingly** and **interesting** help to emphasize the main points and get the attention of the audience.

淡々とデータを説明していくだけの単調な発表だと，どれが重要な情報なのか，聴衆は理解することができない．要点を強調する表現をうまく活用することによって，発表が単調になるのを防ぐことができる．

興味深いことに／面白いことに，〜です.

- **Interestingly,** most of these results show/suggest that temperature rises from day 2.
- **Interestingly,** rates of degradation level off after week 2.
- **It is interesting that** temperature rises from day 2.
- **The interesting point here is that the** temperature rises from day 2.
- **What is interesting (here / in this case / in this experiment) is that** the temperature rises from day 2.

左記の例は，**interestingly**（副詞）や**interesting**（形容詞）を使って要点を示している.

9.4 Using the word note to focus on important information
注目箇所／要点を示すための表現（3）：note

In the following examples, the word **note** is used to focus on important information.

Script(One thing to note is を使って注目してほしい箇所を示す例)

So here we have a lot of data on reliability. <u>One thing to note is</u> the sudden decrease at this point. <u>This indicates</u> a change in the structure of the material.

〜にご注目ください．／注目すべきは〜です．

- <u>One thing to note is</u> the sudden decrease at this point.
- <u>Please note</u> the sudden decrease at this point. <u>This indicates a change in</u> the structure of the material.
- <u>You will note that there is a</u> sudden decrease at this point. <u>This indicates a change in</u> the structure of the material.
- <u>As you have (already) probably noted</u>, there is a sudden decrease at this point. <u>This indicates</u> that the molecules are in an excited state.
- <u>I guess that many of you will have (already) noted that</u> there is a sudden decrease at this point. <u>This shows</u> that the molecules are in an excited state.
- <u>Many of you will have (already) noted that</u> there is a sudden decrease at this point. <u>This means</u> that the molecules are in an excited state.
- <u>Of note is</u> a sudden decrease in reliability. <u>This indicates a change</u> in the structure of the material.

上の例は，動詞 note（注目する／気づく）を使って図表内の注目箇所を示した後，それが何を示しているかを This indicates で説明している．

As you have (already) probably noted や Many of you will have (already) noted that の形で，「皆さんも既にお気づきのとおり」と言うこともできる．

9 Focusing on information on the slide　スライドのどこに注目してほしいかを示す

9.5 How to focus on the main points using the words, stress, emphasize, point out, and draw your attention to
注目箇所／要点を示すための表現(4)：stress, emphasize, point out, draw your attention to

In the examples presented here, the words **stress**, **emphasize**, **point out** and **draw your attention to** are used to focus on the main points.

> Stress, emphasize, point out, draw your attention to はいずれも, 要点を強調したいときに用いる動詞である.

～であることを強調したいと思います．／重要なのは～ということです.

- **I'd like to stress that** although the amount of nutrients in the soil increased, the yield did not decline.
- **I'd like to emphasize that** although the amount of nutrients in the soil increased, the yield did not decline.
- **I'd like to point out that** although the amount of nutrients in the soil increased, the yield did not decline.
- **I want to draw your attention to** the increase in the amount of nutrients in the soil. It means that the yield did not decline.
- **I'd like to draw your attention to** this red line. It shows the yield.
- **I want to draw your attention to the fact that** although the amount of nutrients in the soil increased, the yield did not decline.

Note The expression **draw your attention** to is followed by **to**. Common patterns are **draw your attention to something** and **draw your attention to the fact that**.

- **I want to draw your attention to** figure 1.
- **I'd like to draw your attention to** the increase in temperature.
- **I want to draw your attention to the fact that** the yield did not increase.
- **I'd like to draw your attention to the fact that** the performance improved.

> Draw your attention は I want to / would like to draw your attention to（～に注目してもらいたい）の形で用いられる. 強調したい対象が文章であるときは, to の後ろを the fact that（＋文）として, 「～という事実に注目してもらいたい」の形とする.

148　Part 4 ● How to improve the clarity of the main body　本論を分かりやすく伝える方法

9.6 How to use the words point/points to avoid a flat presentation
注目箇所／要点を示すための表現（5）：point/points

I see a lot of presentations that are generally good, but **too flat**. You can avoid a flat presentation by using these expressions, which focus on key information.

ポイントは，〜ということです．

- **My point is that** after these simple modifications, performance improves dramatically.

● Point　ポイント／要点（単数形）

- **My point is that** after these simple modifications, performance improves dramatically.
- **The point is that** after these simple modifications, performance improves dramatically.
- **The main point is that** after these simple modifications, performance improves dramatically.
- **The key point is that** after these simple modifications, performance improves dramatically.
- **The point I am making is that** after these simple modifications, performance improves dramatically.

● Points　ポイント／要点（複数形）

- **The key points are as follows**. After changes to the system, performance, reliability and speed improved.
- **Here are the key points**. After changes to the system, performance, reliability and speed improved.
- **These are the key points**. After changes to the system, performance, reliability and speed improved.
- **These are the main points**. After changes to the system, performance, reliability and speed improved.

9 Focusing on information on the slide　スライドのどこに注目してほしいかを示す

9.7 How to use the words issue/issues to avoid a flat presentation
注目箇所／要点を示すための表現（6）：issue/issues

～は大きな課題です．

▪ **The main issue is** the stability of the system.

● Issue　課題／問題（単数形）

▪ **The main issue is** the stability of the system.
▪ **So, the biggest issue is** the stability of the system.
▪ **Stability is a big issue** in this field.
▪ **Stability is a big issue** in this type of experiment.
▪ **Another issue is stability.**

● Issues　課題／問題（複数形）

▪ **One of the key issues is** the choice of catalyst.
▪ **There are several issues with** the stability of the system.
▪ **There are a number of issues with** the stability of the system.
▪ **There are several issues here. Reliability, cost and performance.**

Note Presenters sometimes use the following sentence. *This is a big problem.* It is grammatically correct, but a little too direct and somewhat informal. I would change it to, **This is a significant issue** or **This is a serious issue.** The word **issue** is more academic than **problem.** Another frequent error is the use of the following sentences: *That does not matter. It does not matter.* The following sentences are more academic and suitable for a presentation.

▪ **That is not an issue.**
▪ **It is not an issue.**
▪ **Stability is not an issue.**

「大きな問題」を *big problem* とするのはくだけた表現であり，学会発表には相応しくない．Problem ではなく issue を使い，significant issue や serious issue としたほうがよい．

同様に，「問題ではない」を *That does not matter* や *It does not matter* とするのも学会発表では避けたほうがよい．この場合も issue を使って **That is not an issue** などとするのが適切である．

150　Part 4 ● How to improve the clarity of the main body　本論を分かりやすく伝える方法

Focusing on results
結果と考察を説明する

10.1 Signal the start of your explanation of the data using a question
結果の考察を始めることを示す

Here the presenter is moving from description of the results to explanation of them. A question is used to signal the movement from **description** to **explanation**.

この結果は何を意味しているのでしょうか?

- **What do these results mean?**
- **What do these results tell us about** the mechanism?
- **What is the significance of** these results?
- **What can we conclude from** these results?
- **What do these figures tell us about** productivity?
- **What does this graph tell us about** productivity?
- **How can we interpret** this data?

調査・実験の結果を説明する際は,はじめにどのような結果が得られたのかを記述的に説明（description）した後,その結果が何を意味しているか,その結果からどのような結論が導けるか,などの考察を説明（explanation）する. Description から explanation に移る合図として左記のような疑問文を用いると,発表が単調になるのを防ぐことができる.

10.2 Introducing results
結果のまとめを紹介する

Here I show some examples of how to introduce results.

Script（結果のまとめを述べる例）

① So, in this slide, I have summarized the main results I presented in this section. ② With the modified device, using magnesium alloys, we achieved a significant reduction in power consumption. ③ At the same time, we saw an increase in efficiency. ④ In addition, the reliability of the device increased. ⑤ One remaining issue is the difficulty of shaping alloys into new forms. ⑥ We found that through heat treatment, both the microstructure and mechanical properties can be controlled. ⑦ We also noted increases in quality, reliability and strength.

Key sentences

1. Signal that you will introduce the results
結果のまとめを始めることを示す

主な結果のまとめをお示しします.

■ So, **in this slide, I have summarized the main results I presented in this section**.

Examples

■ **Here is a summary of** the main results.

■ **I'll just go over** the main results.

■ **Here I have listed** the key results for this section.

はじめに，結果のまとめが表示されたスライドを示しながら左記のように言うとよい.

152　**Part 4 ● How to improve the clarity of the main body**　本論を分かりやすく伝える方法

2. State results 1 　結果を述べる（1）

〜という結果を得ました.

▌ With the modified device, using magnesium alloys, <u>we achieved a significant reduction in power consumption</u>.

Examples

▌ <u>We obtained</u> a significant reduction <u>in power consumption</u>.

▌ <u>We got</u> a significant reduction <u>in power consumption</u>.

▌ <u>There was</u> a significant reduction <u>in power consumption</u>.

> 「結果を得た」を表す動詞は achieved や obtained が一般的であり, got を使うとややくだけた印象を与える. 一番下の例文のように, There was で表すのも簡単でよい.

The verbs <u>achieved</u> and <u>obtained</u> are formal. The verb <u>got</u> is informal. The last example has a simple pattern. <u>There was</u> a significant reduction in power.

3. State results 2 　結果を述べる（2）

また, 〜という結果も得られました.

▌ <u>At the same time</u>, <u>we saw an increase in efficiency</u>.

Examples

▌ <u>We also observed</u> an increase in efficiency.

▌ <u>There was also</u> an increase in efficiency.

▌ <u>Another thing we saw was that</u> performance improved.

> 追加で結果を述べる際は at the same time（同時に）や also, in addition を用いる. Another thing we saw/noted was と表すこともできる.

10 Focusing on results　結果と考察を説明する　153

4. Additional results　さらに結果を述べる

さらに，〜もみられました.

❚ **In addition, the reliability of the device increased**.

> **Examples**

❚ **There was also** an increase in reliability.

❚ **Another thing we noted** was an increase in reliability.

❚ **Another thing we saw** was an increase in reliability.

5. Refer to issues　課題に言及する

残る課題は，〜です.

❚ **One remaining issue is** the difficulty of shaping alloys into new forms.

> **Examples**

❚ **An outstanding issue is** the difficulty of shaping alloys into new forms.

❚ **Another issue is** the difficulty of shaping alloys into new forms.

❚ **We are still working on** the issue of shaping alloys into new forms.

❚ **One problem is** the difficulty of shaping alloys into new forms.

既に述べた結果（**2〜4**で説明した結果）では解決できていない課題に言及する.「課題／問題」は通常 issue で表す.

154　Part 4 ● How to improve the clarity of the main body　本論を分かりやすく伝える方法

6. Refer to solution　課題の解決策に言及する

～することにより，～できました．

▌ **We found that through heat treatment,** both the microstructure and mechanical properties can be controlled.

Examples

▌ **Through heat treatment, we can control** the microstructure and mechanical properties.

▌ **It is possible to control** the microstructure and mechanical properties using heat treatment.

▌ **We got around** this problem by using heat treatment to control properties.

▌ **We got over** this problem by using heat treatment to control properties.

5 で挙げた課題の解決策を示す．Through ～, we can ～（～によって～できた）の形や，句動詞 get around, get over（ともに「乗り越える」「克服する」という意味をもつ）を用いて表現する．

7. Additional results　さらに結果を述べる

さらに，～もみられました．

▌ **We also noted increases in** quality, reliability and strength.

Examples

▌ **There were also increases in** quality, reliability, and strength.

10 Focusing on results　結果と考察を説明する　155

10.3 Stating that data is not included
含まれていないデータがあることを示す

In some cases, you will need to state that data is not included.

～のデータは含まれておりません.

- That is the data from experiments 1 and 2. We actually did one other experiment, <u>but that data is not included here</u>.
- <u>That data is not included</u>.
- <u>I did not include that data</u>.
- <u>That data is not shown</u>.
- <u>There were some other results that I have not included here</u>.
- <u>There was/were some other data that I have not included here</u>.

結果を示す図表に一部のデータが含まれていないこともある. その場合は左記のように説明するとよい.

10.4 When the reason for something is unknown or unclear: Using the expressions We don't know why, We are not sure why, We don't know the reason for, The reason for X is not clear, The reason for X is unclear   原因がはっきりしないことを示す

In some cases, you will not be able to explain something. Here are some useful expressions.

～の原因ははっきりしません.

- <u>We (still) don't know why</u> the reaction was unsuccessful.
- <u>We are not sure why</u> the reaction was unsuccessful.
- <u>We are not sure why there was</u> a sudden increase in temperature.
- <u>We don't know the reason for</u> the sudden increase in temperature.

結果の考察においては, なぜそのような結果が得られたのかを説明することが必要である. 原因を説明できない場合には, 左記のように述べるとよい.

156　Part 4 ● How to improve the clarity of the main body　本論を分かりやすく伝える方法

- **The reason for** the sudden increase in temperature **is not clear**.
- **The reason for** the sudden increase in temperature **is unclear**.

10.5 Stating that research on a topic is ongoing: Using the verbs checking, looking at, working on, investigating
研究が継続中であることを述べる

In this example, the presenter starts by saying that the reason for something is unknown, and then states that research on the topic is ongoing.

〜の原因は分かりません．この点については現在研究を進めています．

- We are not sure why the reaction was unsuccessful. **We are still checking** that point.
- We are not sure why the reaction was unsuccessful. **We are still looking at** that issue.
- We are not sure why the reaction was unsuccessful. **We are still working on** that issue.
- We are not sure why the reaction was unsuccessful. **We are still investigating** that issue/point.

原因を明らかにするために研究を行っているところである場合は，そのことを現在進行形で示すとよい．

Other reasons for not being able to explain something.

〜の原因は分かりません．それは今回の結果が〜だったからです．

- We don't know the reason for that. **Results were inconclusive**.
- We don't know the reason for that. **Results were difficult to interpret**.
- We can't give a concrete figure. **Results were mixed**.
- We can't really say anything about that issue. **Results were not significant**.

左記のように，原因を説明できない理由を示してもよい［例：inconclusive（この結果からは結論は出せない），difficult to interpret（結果の解釈が困難である），mixed（相反する結論を示す結果が混在している），not significant（有意差が得られなかった）］

10 Focusing on results　結果と考察を説明する

10.6 Giving a reason: Using due to, because of, caused by, the reason for, the result of
原因を説明する

In many cases, it will be necessary to explain why something happens. Here are some examples:

Script(どのような結果が得られたか → その原因は何か, の順に説明する例)

As you can see, there was an increase in temperature on day 4 of the experiment. This was due to interaction between molecules.

● **due to, because of, caused by**

❚ This was because of interaction between molecules.
❚ This was caused by interaction between molecules.

原因をはっきりと説明できる場合には, 左記のいずれかの表現を使って説明する.

● **The reason for**

❚ The reason for this was interaction between molecules.

● **The result of, a result of, as a result of**

❚ This was the result of interaction between molecules.
❚ This was a result of interaction between molecules.
❚ This was as a result of interaction between molecules.

The result of, a result of, as a result of はほぼ同じ意味である.

Note The expressions the result of, a result of, as a result of have the same meaning, but the grammatical patterns are slightly different.

158   Part 4 ● How to improve the clarity of the main body   本論を分かりやすく伝える方法

Common errors──よくある間違い

✗ *The reason of* the increase in temperature is interaction between molecules.

◯ The reason <u>for</u> the increase in temperature is interaction between molecules.

The correct preposition to use with the word **reason** is **for**. You cannot say *The reason of*. The correct pattern is as follows: **The reason for X is Y**.

> 「〜の結果」を *The reason of* とするのは誤りである. *Reason* の後ろに続く前置詞は *of* ではなく **for** であることに注意する.

10.7 Giving a possible reason for something using the expressions: We think that, / We guess that, 考えられる原因を述べる

Here, the presenter states that the <u>reason is not known</u>, but also <u>gives a possible explanation</u> that is introduced with the expressions <u>we think that</u> or <u>we guess that</u>. The sentence has two steps.

1. <u>We don't know the reason for X</u>
2. <u>but we think it was due to Y</u>.

This sentence pattern can be particularly useful in the question and answer session when handling a difficult question.

10 Focusing on results　結果と考察を説明する　159

〜の原因は分かりませんが，私達は〜によるものではない かと考えています.

▌ **We don't know the reason for** the difficulties in shaping alloys into new forms, **but we think that it was due to** a lack of heat control.

● We think that it was due to / We think that it was because of

▌ **We don't know the reason for** the difficulties in shaping alloys into new forms, **but we think that it was due to** a lack of heat control.

▌ **We don't know the reason for** the difficulties in shaping alloys into new forms, **but we think that it was because of** a lack of heat control.

● We guess that it was due to / We guess that it was because of

▌ **We don't know the reason for** the difficulties in shaping alloys into new forms, **but we guess that it was due to** a lack of heat control.

▌ **We don't know the reason for** the difficulties in shaping alloys into new forms, **but we guess that it was because of** a lack of heat control.

▌ **We are not sure why this happened**, **but we guess that it was due to** a buildup of pressure.

▌ **We are not sure why** the sample degraded, **but we guess that it was due to** exposure to sunlight. **There may have been other reasons**.

> **Note** In the last example, the presenter uses the sentence, **There may have been other reasons**. A similar sentence is **That's one possible reason**.

はっきりとは言えない が考えられる原因はあ る，という場合には，左 記のように「原因は分 かりません」→ but → 「〜だと考えます（we think/guess that）」の 形で説明するとよい. この方法は質疑応答の 際に特に有効である.

最後の例文のように， 「（〜だと考えます.）し かし他の原因もあり得 ます」と言いたいとき は，There may have been other reasons と すればよい. 同じよう な意味で That's one possible reason（これ はあくまで1つの可能 性です）と言うことも できる.

10.8 Speculating on the reason for something using probably, because of, one possible reason is, one possible explanation is, perhaps　原因を推測する：確信の度合いを下げるための表現

Here the presenter gives possible reasons for something, but uses less direct language such as **probably**, **because of**, **one possible reason is**, **one possible explanation is** and **perhaps**.

~の原因はおそらく~です．

- The reason for the sudden increase in temperature was probably the increased reaction time.

● Probably　おそらく

- The reason for the sudden increase in temperature was probably the increased reaction time.
- The sudden increase in temperature was probably because of the addition of another catalyst.
- The sudden increase in temperature was probably as a result of the reduction in the number of samples.
- The sudden increase in temperature was probably due to the reduction in the number of samples.

● Because of　~の原因により

- We don't know the reason for this. It might be because of the number of samples. Another reason might be the size of the samples.

● One possible reason is　考えられる原因の1つは~

- We don't know why the samples cracked. One possible reason is the higher temperature.

推測された原因を述べる際は，必要に応じて確信の度合いを下げる表現（probably など）を使い，「はっきりとは分からない」ことを聴衆に強調するようにする．

10 Focusing on results　結果と考察を説明する　161

● **One possible explanation is** 考えられる説明の１つは〜

■ We aren't sure why the experiment failed. One possible explanation is a buildup of pressure in the system.

■ We aren't sure why the experiment failed. One possible explanation is an increase of pressure in the system.

● **Perhaps** もしかすると

■ Perhaps something happened in the central nervous system. We really don't know at the moment. We are still working on that.

In this example, there are three steps. First, the presenter offers a possible reason for something. Perhaps something happened in the central nervous system. Next, it is stated that the reason is unknown. We really don't know at the moment. Finally, it is stated that further research work is being conducted on this issue. We are still working on that.

左記の例文は,「もしかすると〜かもしれません」→「しかし,実際のところは現時点ではまだ分かりません」→「この点については現在も研究を進めています」の３段階で説明している.

10.9 **When you cannot explain something, refer to future work**
説明が難しいときの対応 (1)：今後の研究に言及する

When they cannot explain why something happens, some presenters **refer to future work**.

〜の原因は分かりません．この点については今後の研究を予定しています．

■ We are not sure why this happens. We are planning to do further experiments on this issue.

■ We are not sure of the cause of the problem. We are carrying out more experiments on this issue.

■ We don't know the reason for this issue. We are still working on it.

現時点のデータでは説明が難しい内容については,「〜については現在調査中です／今後の研究を予定しています」のように述べることもできる.

162　　Part 4 ● How to improve the clarity of the main body　本論を分かりやすく伝える方法

10.10 Using the word basically to explain something simply
説明が難しいときの対応(2)：単純化して説明する

The word basically is a useful way of giving a short, simple explanation.

〜について説明するのは難しいのですが，簡単に言うと〜です．

- I'm not sure how to describe it. Basically, it is a 2-step reaction with the addition of a catalyst.
- I'm not sure how to explain it. Basically, it is a 2-step reaction with the addition of a catalyst.
- It's difficult to explain. Basically, it is a 2 step-reaction with the addition of a catalyst.

厳密な説明，正確な説明を行うのが難しい場合には，basically（簡単に言うと／基本的には）を文頭に置いて，単純化／簡略化された説明を行うようにする．

Introducing references
参考文献を示す／結果を先行研究と比較する

Here I give examples of how to introduce references and URLs.

 11.1 Referring to references on your slides with the following words and expressions: here, check, check out, look at, take a look at, describe, description, find, see　参考文献を示す

I have noticed that more presenters are including references on their slides. Here, I give examples of how to introduce them. Please remember to use the pointer to draw the attention of the audience to the reference / references.

> 口頭発表では，スライドに参考文献リストを表示し，詳細についてはそちらを参照するように伝えることも多い．

Script（詳細の説明は省き，参考文献を参照するように伝える例）

This slide shows the experimental setup. I'll skip the exact details of the apparatus. If you are interested, <u>here are the references</u>, which give a detailed explanation of the apparatus.

興味のある方は，こちらの参考文献をご参照ください．

- If you are interested, <u>here are the references</u>, which give a detailed explanation of the apparatus.

● **Here**
- <u>Here are the references</u>.
- <u>Here are the relevant references</u>.

● **Check**
- <u>Please check this reference / these references</u>.
- <u>If you want to see the details, please check this reference / these references</u>.

> Here を使う場合は，スライド内の参考文献リストをレーザーポインターで指しながら「こちらが参考文献です」のように言う．

> Check や check out，look at，take a look at を使う場合は，「こちらの参考文献をご確認ください」のように言う．

164　Part 4 ● How to improve the clarity of the main body　本論を分かりやすく伝える方法

Check out

- **If you are interested in the details, please check out this reference / these references**.

Look at

- **If you want to see the details, please look at** this reference / these references.

Take a look at

- **If you are interested in the details, please take a look at this reference** / **these references**.

Describe

- The system / setup / approach **is described in detail in this reference**.
- The system / setup / approach **is described here**.

Description

- **This reference contains a detailed description of** the experimental set up.
- **There is a description of the method in this reference**.

Find

- **You can find a detailed explanation of this process here**.

See

- **You can see the details in this reference / these references**.
- **You can see our other work here**.
- **You can see our other work in these references**.
- **You can see that approach in these references**.

Describe（動詞）や description（名詞）を使う場合は、「～についてはこちらの参考文献に記載されています」「こちらの文献には～についての詳しい記述がございます」のような表現になる.

Find や see を使う場合は、「～についての詳しい説明はこちらの参考文献でご覧になれます」のように言う.

Ⅱ Introducing references　参考文献を示す／結果を先行研究と比較する

11.2 How to refer to URLs
参考 URL を示す

In addition to referring to references, you might want to draw people's attention to URLs that contain relevant information.

Script(参考 URL について説明する例)

> So these are the main areas of research that we cover at our institute. A more detailed explanation can be found in this URL.

こちらの URL をご参照ください.
- I've included some relevant URLs here.
- Here are some useful URLs.
- You might find these URLs useful.
- If you are interested, please check these URLs.

ウェブサイトの URL を紹介するときは左記のように言うとよい.

11.3 How to use the expression in the literature
結果を先行研究と比較する：in the literature の使い方

It is important to put your data in the context of results in the same field. For that reason, presenters compare their findings to what has been reported elsewhere. The phrase **in the literature** is frequently used. Here are some examples.

Script(実験の結果と先行研究で報告されている値を比較する例)

> So, as you can see from the results, we obtained a yield of 5 to 6 percent. Similar yields are reported in the literature.

Part 4 ● How to improve the clarity of the main body　本論を分かりやすく伝える方法

先行研究／文献では，〜と報告されています．

▌ Similar yields are reported <u>in the literature</u>.

Examples

▌ <u>In the literature,</u> reported values are in the region of 5 to 6 percent.

▌ Reported values <u>in the literature</u> are in the region of 5 to 6 percent.

▌ This means that our results <u>are in line with the literature</u>.

Common errors──よくある間違い

✗ *In literature,* values are in the region of 5 to 6 percent.

✗ *In literatures,* values are in the region of 5 to 6 percent.

○ <u>In the literature,</u> values are in the region of 5 to 6 percent.

○ <u>In the literature,</u> average values were in the region of 5 to 6 percent.

In literature, should be <u>in the literature</u>. The word literature is classified as a group or collective noun, and therefore needs a definite article. *In literatures* is incorrect. Literature is not countable and is a collective noun. Generally, the word literature is not plural

✗ *In their literature,* Watanabe reported values are in the region of 5 to 6 percent.

○ <u>Watanabe 2018 reported</u> values in the region of 5 to 6 percent.

This is a reference relating to a specific paper. It is not possible to say *in their literature*. It is better to state the **author** and **year of the paper** in this pattern, <u>Watanabe 2018 reported</u>.

Literature は集合名詞であり，定冠詞 the が必要である．また不可算名詞であるため s はつかない．そのため文献の数にかかわらず常に in the literature の形となることに注意する．

特定の論文を指して「○○らの論文」と言いたいとき，*in their literature* とするのは誤りである．左記のように「著者名＋発表年」の形で示すのがよい．

> ✗ Based on *many literature,* we decided to use a value of 15 percent.
> ○ Based on the literature, we decided to use a value of 15 percent

> Literature は集合名詞であるため、「多い」「少ない」をつけることはできない．

The expression *many literature* is incorrect because literature is a collective noun and is generally singular.

 11.4　Other expressions using the word literature
文献に関するその他の表現

Here are some more examples that use the word literature.

> この結果は先行研究で報告されている結果と一致しています．
>
> - This means that our results are <u>in line with reported values in the literature</u>.
> - This means that our results are <u>in line with the literature</u>.
> - This means that our results are <u>much the same as those reported in the literature</u>.
> - These results are <u>pretty similar to what is in the literature</u>.
> - This result is <u>consistent with what is in the literature</u>.

> 研究結果が先行研究の結果と一致していることを示すには、左記のように in line with, much the same as, pretty similar to, consistent with などを用いる．

> 文献レビューによると，〜です．
>
> - Based <u>on a literature review,</u> we found average yields were in the region of 2 million tons.
> - Based <u>on a review of the literature,</u> we found average yields were in the region of 2 million tons.

12 Summarizing at 3 levels: one slide, several slides, a section
発表の途中にまとめを挟む：スライド1枚のまとめ，スライド数枚分のまとめ，セクションのまとめ

This section contains sentences that will help you to summarize information at 3 different levels as follows: **one slide**, **several slides**, and **a section**.

Many presenters think that there is only one summary in a presentation, and that it is always at the end of the presentation. In fact, during a presentation, you will probably want to **give several mini-summaries**, **in addition to** a summary at the end of the presentation. These mini-summaries can be at the level of **one slide**, **several slides** or **a section**.

まとめを発表全体の最後にしか行わない発表者も多いが，聴衆の理解を助けるためには，発表の途中にもそれまでの内容のまとめを挟むと効果的である．

本項では，(1) スライド1枚の内容のまとめ，(2) スライド数枚分の内容のまとめ，(3) セクションのまとめ，の3段階のまとめの述べ方を紹介する．

12.1 Summarizing one slide
まとめを述べる(1)：スライド1枚のまとめ

It is not necessary to summarize the information presented in every slide, but if a slide has a lot of data or is particularly important, it will help the audience if you can briefly stress the main points in the form of a short summary. In some cases, the main point or points will be presented at the bottom of the slide. In the example below, the expression, **the substrate is thinner and more flexible**, can be positioned at the bottom of the slide.

In most cases, summarizing a single slide will be in the form of a main point or points, or some kind of take-home message. Here are some examples.

全てのスライドでまとめを述べる必要はないが，特に情報量が多いスライドや重要なスライドについては，一言まとめを述べると聴衆の理解に役立つ．その際，口頭でまとめを述べるのに加えて，スライドの最下部にまとめの1文を入れるのもよい．

次ページの例の場合，スライド下部に入れるまとめの1文は, the substrate is thinner and more flexible となる．スライド下部のまとめ文のつくり方については，pp. 96〜98 を参照．

このスライドのポイントは，〜ということです．

- **The key point/issue here is that** the substrate is thinner and more flexible.
- **The thing to remember here is that** the substrate is thinner and more flexible.
- **So, the main point in this slide is that** the substrate is thinner and more flexible.
- **The main message here is that** the substrate is thinner and more flexible.
- **The take-home message from this data is that** the substrate is thinner and more flexible.

> (Note) The expression **the take-home message is** can be used to summarize data in **a single slide**, **a section**, as well as in **a summary slide** at the end of the presentation.

最後の例文は take-home message（テイクホームメッセージ＝聴衆に家に持って帰ってもらいたいメッセージ）という表現を使っている．この表現は，発表全体のまとめを述べる際だけでなく，スライド1枚のまとめやスライド数枚分のまとめを述べる際にも使うことができる．

12.2 Summarizing several slides
まとめを述べる(2)：スライド数枚分のまとめ

To summarize the main points from several slides, presenters use a 2-step system as follows: **1. Signal the start of the summary 2. Briefly list the main points**. Here are some examples.

スライド数枚分のまとめを述べるには，①まとめを始める合図→②要点をいくつか述べる，の2段階で行う．

ここでいったん，ここまでの数枚のスライドのまとめをいたします．ポイントは〜です．

- **We have covered quite a lot of ground. So I'd like to summarize** what we have seen in the last few slides. （short summary of the main points）
- **I'd like to summarize what we have seen in the last few slides**. The main points are （short summary of the main points）
- **This is what we have seen in the last few slides**. （short summary of the main points）

「ここまでの数枚のスライド」は last few slides で表す．

170　Part 4 ● How to improve the clarity of the main body　本論を分かりやすく伝える方法

12.3 Summarizing a section
まとめを述べる（3）：セクションのまとめ

このセクションのまとめをいたします．ポイントは〜です．

- **I'd like to wrap up this section by summarizing the main points.**（short summary of the main points）
- **I'd just like to summarize the main points in this section.**（short summary of the main points）
- **I'll just go over** the main points in this section.（short summary of the main points）
- **I'll just run through** the main points from this section.（short summary of the main points）
- **The take-home message for this section is** as follows.（short summary of the main points）
- **These are the main points from this section.**（short summary of the main points）

まとめを述べることを示すには，wrap up, go over, run through などの句動詞を使うと便利である．これらの句動詞については part 5 の pp. 188〜190 も参照．

⑫ Summarizing at 3 levels: one slide, several slides, a section
発表の途中にまとめを挟む：スライド1枚のまとめ，スライド数枚分のまとめ，セクションのまとめ

From data to explanation and implications
結果を考察する：結果が何を意味しているか／どのような意義をもつか

A lot of time will be spent **introducing data and results**. For the audience to be able to process what is presented, the presenter will need to **explain the meaning of the data**, and **the implications**.

研究の結果の説明にあたっては，単にどのような結果が得られたかを述べるだけではなく，その結果がどのような意味をもつか，学術的・応用的にどのような意義をもつかなどについて考察することも必要である．

Here is an example.

Script（どのような結果か → 何を意味しているか → どのような意義をもつか，の順に説明する例）

> **The data shows** an increase in temperature and reaction speed. **This means that** molecules are excited and move freely. **In terms of manufacturing**, we can fabricate thinner, more flexible films.

13.1 Introduce the data on the slide
どのような結果であるかを紹介する

The following examples are simple statements of what is on the slide.

この結果から〜ということが読み取れます．

- **The data shows** an increase in temperature and reaction speed.
- **As you can see** from the data I have presented, there is an increase in temperature and reaction speed.
- **What we have seen from this data is that** there is an increase in temperature and reaction speed.

結果を示す図表から何が読み取れるか（例：数値の上昇）を説明する際は，左記のような表現を用いる．

172　Part 4 ● How to improve the clarity of the main body　本論を分かりやすく伝える方法

13.2 Explain the data
結果が何を意味しているかを説明する

Here the presenter gives an explanation of the data presented using the expressions, **This means that**, **This suggests that**, **So these results tell us that**.

この結果は，〜ということを意味しています．

- **This means** that molecules are excited and move freely.
- **This suggests** that molecules are excited and move freely.
- **So, these results tell us** that molecules are excited and move freely.

13.1 で説明した結果がどのような意味をもっているかについては、**This means that** や **This suggests that**, **So, these results tell us that** などを使って説明する.

13.3 Explain the implications
結果のもつ意義を説明する

At this point. the presenter comments on how the data affects the wider picture, which in this case is the manufacturing process.

○○分野において，
この結果がもつ意義は／与える影響は〜です．

- **In terms of** manufacturing, we can fabricate thinner more flexible films.
- **The main implications for the manufacturing process are that** thinner and more flexible films can be obtained.
- **So, what this means is that** we are able to manufacture more flexible films.
- **So, the important point here is that** we can manufacture thinner and more flexible films.

この研究の結果が他の研究にどのような影響を与えるか，あるいはどのような応用的意義を有するかを説明するには，左記のように言う.

In terms of を使って，「○○分野において〜」の部分を明確に示すとよい.

The presenter brings in the wider picture using the expressions **in terms of** and **the main implications are** to introduce the point.

13 From data to explanation and implications
結果を考察する：結果が何を意味しているか／どのような意義をもつか

173

Introducing and explaining a video clip
動画を再生する

The number of presenters using short video clips in their presentations has increased, but simply showing a video clip is not enough. The presenter needs **to support the video clip with appropriate English**. Below I have listed several useful sentences.

口頭発表で動画を活用するのは効果的であるが，ただ単に動画を流すだけでは不十分で，動画のどこがポイントなのか，口頭で適宜補足説明を加えるのが重要である．

14.1 Introducing a video clip
これから再生する動画を紹介する

これから〜の動画をお見せします．

- **I'm going to show you a short video of** the catalytic conversion.
- **I'd like to show you a video clip of** the reaction.
- **I'm going to show you a video clip of** the reaction.
- **I have a video clip of** the reaction that I'm going to show you.
- **This is a video clip of** the reaction.

はじめに，何についての動画を再生するのか，1文で簡単に説明する．

Common errors——よくある間違い

- ✗ Please *look at* the video.
- ✗ Please *watch* this video.
- ◯ **I'm going to show you a video clip of** the reaction.
- ◯ **This is a video clip of the reaction**.

The expressions *please look at* and *please watch* are incorrect. Better expressions are as follows: I'd like to show you a video clip. I'm going to show you a video clip. This is a video clip of the reaction.

動画を再生する際に *please look at* や *please watch* と言うのは誤りである．この場合，*I'd like to show you a video clip* などと言うことが多い．

174　Part 4 ● How to improve the clarity of the main body　本論を分かりやすく伝える方法

14.2 Describing a number of stages in a process or reaction
動画の各段階について説明する

Script(動画の各段階の説明 → 動画のまとめ，の順に説明する例)

① <u>At this point</u>, the sample is stable and there is no reaction. ② <u>Here you can see</u> the first stages of the reaction. The edge of the sample is changing color. ③ <u>This is followed by</u> combustion. ④ <u>Finally</u>, the sample becomes hard. ⑤ <u>So, what is the significance of the chemical reaction?</u> <u>I think we have seen that</u> the reaction is stable. ⑥ <u>This means that</u> the process has various possible applications.

Key sentences

1. Start the explanation　現象が始まる前の状態を説明する

この時点では，〜です．

- <u>At this point</u>, the sample is stable and there is no reaction.

Examples

- <u>At this stage</u>, the sample is stable and there is no reaction.
- <u>Here,</u> the sample is stable and there is no reaction.
- <u>So, in the beginning,</u> the sample is stable and there is no reaction.

学会発表で動画を再生する場合，何らかの現象（例：化学反応）の一部始終を捉えたものであることが多い．その場合，現象の各段階について，今何が起こっているのかを口頭で説明するとよい．

はじめに，動画の再生開始時点（現象が始まる前）の状態を説明する．「この時点では」は **At this point** などで表す．

14 Introducing and explaining a video clip　動画を再生する

175

2. Move on to the next stage　最初に起こる変化を説明する

ご覧のとおり，～が始まりました.

■ <u>Here you can see</u> the first stages of the reaction.

Examples

■ <u>As you can see,</u> these are the first stages of the reaction.
■ <u>Here we can observe</u> the initial stages of the reaction quite clearly.
■ <u>So, this is the start of the first stages of the reaction</u>.

現象が始まったことを示すには左記のように言う.「ご覧のとおり，（今現象が始まりました）」は Here you can see や As you can see で表す.

3. Introduce the following stage　次の状態を説明する

続いて，～が起こります.

■ <u>This is followed by</u> combustion.

Examples

■ <u>And next,</u> the sample catches on fire.
■ <u>After that,</u> we get combustion.
■ <u>At this point,</u> combustion takes place.
■ <u>And now,</u> combustion takes place.

次に起こる現象については左記のように説明する. A is followed by B は「A に続いて B が起こる」を表す.

4. Explain the last stage　最終的な状態を説明する

最終的には，～となります.

■ <u>Finally,</u> the sample becomes hard.

Examples

■ <u>This is the last stage of the reaction</u>. And the sample becomes hard.
■ <u>The sample is hard</u>.
■ <u>The sample becomes hard</u>.
■ <u>In the end,</u> the sample becomes hard.
■ <u>By the time the reaction finishes,</u> the sample becomes hard.

動画の終わり（現象の終了後）の状態を説明して，動画の再生を終える.

176　**Part 4 ● How to improve the clarity of the main body**　本論を分かりやすく伝える方法

14.3 Signal the start of the explanation
動画のポイントを説明することを示す

この動画のポイントは何でしょうか？

- <u>So, what is the significance of</u> the chemical reaction?

Examples

- <u>We have seen various stages of the reaction</u>. <u>The question is, what is the significance of it</u>?

> 動画を再生した後は，動画のどの点が重要であったのかを述べ，動画のまとめを行う．はじめに，説明を始める合図として左記のように言う．

14.4 Concluding the video sequence with an explanation
ポイントを述べて動画の説明を終える

この動画のポイントは，〜ということです．このことは〜を意味します．

- <u>I think we have seen that</u> the reaction is stable. <u>This means that</u> the process has various possible applications.

Examples

- <u>What we have seen is that</u> the reaction has 4 stages.
- <u>So, this shows that</u> the reaction is stable, <u>and can be applied to</u> various industrial processes.
- <u>I think we have seen the reaction is stable</u>. <u>This means it can be controlled</u>.
- <u>This means that</u> the process can be used industrially for a variety of uses.

> 動画で示した内容の何が重要であったか，それが何を意味しているかについて説明する．

14 Introducing and explaining a video clip　動画を再生する

Time management, correcting yourself, correcting an error on a slide
発表時間の管理／発言内容とスライド内容の訂正

Here I include some useful expressions concerning **time issues**, **how to correct yourself** and **dealing with an error on the slide**.

15.1 Time management
発表時間の管理

If you think you don't have enough time left, you can use these sentences.

> 時間がありませんので，〜に移ります／〜は省略します．
>
> ■ **I'm running out of time. So, I'll move on to** the discussion section.
> ■ **Since time is short, I'll go straight to** the summary.
> ■ **I don't have much time left, so I'll skip these slides**.

発表時間をオーバーしそうなとき，時間短縮のために一部の内容を飛ばす場合は左記のように言う．スライドを飛ばすときの表現については，(p. 132) も参照．

If you spoke over the time limit, you can use this sentence.

> 申し訳ありません．1，2分オーバーしてしまいました．
>
> ■ **Sorry. I think I went over by a minute or two**.

発表時間をオーバーしてしまった場合の謝罪は左記のようになる．「(時間を) オーバーする」は **go over** (by+時間) で表す．

178　Part 4 ● How to improve the clarity of the main body　本論を分かりやすく伝える方法

15.2 Correcting yourself
発言内容を訂正する

In some cases, you will need to correct what you have just said. For example, you might have misread a number or said something incorrectly.

失礼しました. ××ではなく○○です.

- **Excuse me, I meant to say** 150 not 250.
- **I'm sorry. I should have said that** temperature increased not decreased.

口頭での説明を言い間違えた場合は, 左記のように訂正する. 謝罪→訂正の順で, 謝罪はExcuse me か I'm sorry, 訂正は I meant to say / should have said (＋正しい内容) not (＋誤った内容) のように言うとよい.

15.3 Correcting an error on a slide
スライドの内容を訂正する

すみません. スライドに誤りがありました. ××ではなく○○です.

- **I've just seen a mistake on this slide. The title should be** degradable **not** non-degradable.
- **Excuse me, that number should be** 179 **not** 197.
- **I'm sorry. That should be** 179.
- **Excuse me. That should read** 179.
- **Sorry that's a mistake. It should be** 179 **not** 197.

スライドの内容の誤りに気づいた場合は, 左記のように that should be (＋正しい内容) not (＋誤った内容) のように訂正する.

16 How to use the expressions stand for and is short for to introduce an acronym
アクロニム（頭字語）を説明する

In the example below, the acronym is AIST and the full title is introduced with the 2-word verb **stands for**. Another expression that you can use is, **is short for**

> ○○（アクロニム）は〜の略です．
>
> ■ AIST <u>stands for</u> Advanced Institute of Science and Technology.
> ■ AIST <u>is short for</u> Advanced Institute of Science and Technology.

Acronym（アクロニム）とは日本語で「頭字語」のことで，先頭の文字をつなげて１つの単語となったもののことである．

アクロニムの説明には**stands for** または **is short for** のいずれかを用いる．この場合 *mean* は使えないことに注意する．

> ### Common errors──よくある間違い
>
> ✕ AIST, *in short*, Advanced Institute of Science and Technology.
> ✕ AIST, *shortly*, Advanced Institute of Science and Technology.
> ✕ AIST, *short for*, Advanced Institute of Science and Technology.
> ✕ AIST, *means*, Advanced Institute of Science and Technology.
> ○ AIST **stands for** Advanced Institute of Science and Technology.
> ○ AIST **is short for** Advanced Institute of Science and Technology.

The above errors should be changed to <u>stands for</u> or <u>is short for</u>. These expressions have the same meaning. Please note that the word *means* cannot be used to introduce an acronym.

7 Giving examples using such as, for example, for instance

具体例を挙げて説明する

> **Script**(for example の後ろに続けて利点の具体例を挙げている例)
>
> Although amalgam has traces of mercury, it does have several advantages, <u>for example</u> hardness, durability and cost.

I'm surprised that presenters fail to give examples, especially when a simple example would help the audience to understand the point being made. Here I introduce three of the most frequently used expressions for introducing examples.

聴衆の理解を助けるため，なるべく具体例を挙げて説明するとよい．具体例を口頭で述べる際は，**such as** や **for example**，**for instance** を用いる．

たとえば○○（具体例）です．／○○（具体例）などの〜．

- The samples should be treated with some kind of nucleophile, <u>**such as**</u> alcohol or ether.
- The system is susceptible to factors <u>**such as**</u> moisture, temperature and vibration.
- This was calculated using variables <u>**such as**</u> speed, weight and mass.
- I'll just quickly mention some possible applications. The system can be used in various ways, **such as / for example / for instance**, medical applications.

17.1 How to introduce an example. Referring to material on the slide you are currently showing
スライドに具体例を表示させる(1)：現在のスライド

Here I show how to introduce examples with the expressions: **This is**, **Here we have**, **Here are**, **I'll show you**, **I'll give you**.

たとえばこのような例があります．

- **This is an example**.
- **This is an example of the reaction process**.
- **This is a typical example**.
- **Here we have a typical example**.
- **Here are some examples**.

口頭で例を挙げるだけではなく，具体例をスライドに表示させて説明することもできる．現在のスライドに具体例が示されている場合には，左記のように述べるとよい．

17.2 How to introduce an example when referring to material on the next slide
スライドに具体例を表示させる(2)：次のスライド

具体例は次のスライドでお示しします．

- **I'll show you an example** in the next slide / later.
- **I'll show you some examples** in the next slide.
- **I'll give you some examples of** that in the next slide.
- **I'll introduce some examples of** the system in the next section.

具体例を次のスライドで示すことを予告する場合は，左記のように言う．

8 Explaining a process using the words first, next, after that, then

手順を説明する

In this example, the presenter uses **first**, **next**, **after that**, and **then** to explain a process. This is a standard way of sequencing a number of steps.

> **はじめに～を行いました．次に～して，最後に～しました.**
>
> ▍ <u>First,</u> the samples were washed. <u>Next,</u> they were dried. <u>After that</u> they were stored. **Then** we calculated the difference in weight.

実験の手順などを説明する際は，first, next, after that, then などの順序を表す表現を活用するとよい.

It is also possible to reduce the length of the sentence by deleting the words **first**, **next**, **after that**, and **then**.

> ▍ <u>We washed, dried and stored the samples</u>. <u>Then, we calculated</u> the difference in weight.

左記のように，順序を表す単語を減らし，より簡潔な文にすることもできる.

18 Explaining a process using the words first, next, after that, then　手順を説明する　183

Column #04

Is it okay to read from the text on your computer?
口頭発表で原稿を読み上げるのは問題か？

Nowadays, computers are equipped with a handy tool that means you can write the script for your presentation at the bottom of the screen and read from it. Some presenters ask me if this okay. Personally, I do not think this is a problem. As you are speaking, the audience will be busy looking at the slides and listening to your explanation, and no one will notice that you are reading from a script. There is, however, one problem. Because you are reading from the computer screen, your presentation may appear to be flat and rather monotonous. You can avoid this problem if you have a script that is informal and uses spoken English, not formal, written English. Of course, it would be better if you could give a presentation without a script, but for many presenters this is too difficult. Reading from the script is acceptable and is one step on the way to giving a presentation without notes.

原稿を読み上げると，発表が単調になってしまいやすい．原稿を使わずに発表するのが理想ではあるが，それが難しい場合は，話し言葉の英語を活用することで発表が単調になるのを回避することができる．

Part 5
Finishing your presentation
発表の終わり方

In this part of the book, I introduce a 16-step guide for finishing your presentation. The focus is on useful sentences and vocabulary that will help you to give a clear and concise summary of the main points of your presentation.

　発表の終わりには，発表内容の要点を簡潔に振り返った後，聴衆へのお礼を述べて発表を締めくくります．本章では，発表の終わり方の流れを 16 のステップに分けて紹介します．なお，その際に使用する「まとめスライド」については次章（Part 6）で解説します．

Presentation styles have changed. <u>Previously</u>, presenters signaled the end of their presentation with, <u>In conclusion</u>, and used <u>formal written language</u> such as, <u>It was suggested that</u> or <u>Within the limitations of this study, we could achieve significant improvements in performance</u>. Slides consisted of <u>full sentences</u>, which <u>the presenter read out word for word</u>. In some cases, the presenter said nothing and expected the audience to read what was on the last slide. <u>The last part of the presentation was flat and had little or no impact</u>.

<u>Today</u>, presenters finish their presentations with sentences such as: <u>This is my last slide</u>, <u>This is a summary</u>, <u>This is the take-home message</u>. The final slide consists of <u>a short summary of the main points of the presentation,</u> presented on the slide <u>with bullet points</u>. These are <u>supported by a script using simple English</u>. The English on the slide and the script are different. It is common to <u>mention future research, funding and acknowledgments.</u> The summary slide has <u>become more complex</u>, <u>includes more information</u>, and is <u>a crucial part of the presentation</u>.

・以前の学会発表では，最後のスライドには研究の結論が論文のような文章で記されており，発表者はそれをそのまま読み上げるのが一般的だった．

・最近では，発表内容の要点を箇条書きでまとめたスライドを作成し，それを簡潔な英語で説明することが増えてきた．

Finishing: A 16-step guide for finishing your presentation
発表を締めくくるための 16 ステップ

Starting the summary: Steps 1～5
まとめを始める：ステップ 1～5

1. Signal the start of the summary 〈まとめに入ることを示す〉
2. Remind the audience of your current research 〈現在の研究内容を再度述べる〉
3. Remind the audience of the topic 〈発表テーマを再度述べる〉
4. Restate the objectives 〈研究目的を再度述べる〉
5. Restate research questions 〈疑問・仮説を再度述べる〉

Introduce the findings, additional findings, the main message, the take-home message, implications, and future work: Steps 6～11
研究結果のポイントや聴衆へのメッセージを述べる：ステップ 6～11

6. Introduce the findings 〈結果を紹介する〉
   6.1 Signal the start of the findings
   6.2 Stating the findings
   6.3 Introducing additional findings
7. Explain the findings 〈結果から得られる結論を説明する〉
   7.1 Introduce the start of the explanation
   7.2 Main message
8. State the take-home message 〈テイクホームメッセージを述べる〉
9. Mention the implications 〈研究の意義を述べる〉
10. Finishing 〈まとめを終える〉
11. Mention future work 〈今後の研究課題を述べる〉

Finishing the presentation: Steps 12～16
発表を終える：ステップ 12～16

12. Funding 〈研究助成に言及する〉
13. Acknowledgments 〈謝辞を述べる〉
14. Signal the end of the presentation 〈結びの挨拶を述べる〉
15. Contact details 〈連絡先を紹介する〉
16. Invite questions 〈質問を呼びかける〉

Starting the summary: Steps 1-5
まとめを始める：ステップ 1〜5

1 Signal the start of the summary
まとめに入ることを示す

Here are some examples of how to signal the start of the summary using the words **last**, **finish**, **summary**, **summarize**, **run through**, **go over**, **wrap up**.

はじめに，これからまとめに入ることを 1 文で示す．その際，last, finish, summary, summarize, run through, go over, wrap up のいずれかを用いるとよい（いずれか 1 つで十分であり，複数を組み合わせる必要はない）．

● Last

これが最後のスライドです．

- This is the last slide.
- This is my last slide.

 Both of the following expressions are possible: **the last slide** and **my last slide**.

Last を用いる場合は，「これが最後のスライド（＝まとめスライド）です」のように言う．「最後のスライド」は **the last slide** でも **my last slide** でもどちらでもよい（学会発表では通常 my は用いないが，この場合は使用可能．詳しくは p. 16 のコラムを参照）．

● Finish

最後にまとめを述べて，本日の発表を終えたいと思います．

- I'd like to finish with a summary.
- I'm going to finish by making the following points.
- I want to finish by summarizing the main points / the main findings.
- I want to finish by going over the main points.
- I'm going to finish by reviewing the main points.

Finish を用いる場合は，finish with a summary または finish by 〜ing the main points/findings のいずれかの形となることが多い．

 Frequently used patterns are as follows: **finish with** a summary, **finish by verb+ing**, **summarizing**, **reviewing**, **talking about**, + **the main points, the main findings**.

188　Part 5 ● Finishing your presentation　発表の終わり方

● Summary

こちらが本日の発表のまとめです.

- **This is a summary**.
- **I'd like to finish with a summary**.
- **This is a summary of the main points I made today**.
- **This is a summary of the main points**.
- **This is a summary of the main findings**.
- **This is a summary of the results**.

「まとめを述べる」と言いたい場合, 名詞 summary と動詞 summarize のいずれも使用できる.

● Summarize

本日の発表のまとめを行いたいと思います.

- **I'd like to summarize my presentation**.
- **I'd like to summarize the findings**.
- **I'd like to summarize the main points I made today**.
- **I'm going to summarize this presentation**.
- **I want to summarize the main points**.
- **I'll (quickly) summarize the main points / the most important findings**.

● Run through

本日の発表の要点をおさらいしたいと思います.

- **I'd like to run through the main points I made today**.
- **I'm going to run through the main points**.
- **I'll (just) run through the main points**.

Run through は「要点のみを簡単に説明する」というニュアンスをもつ句動詞である. 3番目の例文の just も同様に「要点のみを簡単に」という意味合いであり, 省略しても構わない.

Note The word just signals that the presenter will briefly explain the main points. It is possible to omit just as the two-word verb run through indicates that what follows is a short summary of the main points.

Starting the summary: Steps 1-5　まとめを始める：ステップ 1〜5

● Go over

本日の発表の要点を振り返りたいと思います.

▌ **I'd like to go over the main points**.
▌ **I want to go over the main findings**.
▌ **I'd like to go over the main points I covered today**.
▌ **I'm going to go over the main findings（in this work/ study/research）**.

> **Note** The verbs <u>run through</u> and <u>go over</u> mean to explain something briefly, and are particularly useful when you have a lot of information but can only focus on the main points.

Go over も run through と同じようなニュアンスをもつ. まとめのように, 多くの情報の中から重要なポイントだけをかいつまんで説明する際に便利な表現である.

● Wrap up

本日の発表のまとめを行いたいと思います.

▌ **I'm going to wrap up this presentation**.
▌ **I'd like to wrap up this presentation with a short summary**.
▌ **I want to wrap up this presentation by talking about the main results and mentioning our future work**.
▌ **I want to wrap up this presentation by going over the main points and talking about future directions**.
▌ **I'm going to wrap up this presentation by reviewing the main points and talking about future directions**.

Wrap up は「まとめる」「仕上げる」「終える」などの意味をもつ句動詞であり, 発表を終える際によく用いられる.

> **Note** Any of the examples in this section, **1. Signal the start of the summary**, can be used alone to start the summary. It is not necessary to combine them. Just one sentence from this section is enough to signal that you will start the summary.

ここまでに紹介した例文はいずれか1つを用いれば十分であり, 複数を組み合わせる必要はない.

190 　Part 5 ● Finishing your presentation　発表の終わり方

2 Remind the audience of your current research interests
現在の研究内容を再度述べる

Some presenters **briefly refer to their current research interests**. In most cases, this is just a single sentence.

まとめの最初に，自分がどのような研究を行っているかを簡単に振り返る発表者もいる．

私達は〜についての研究を行っています．

- **We have been working on** ways of reducing energy loss in this device.
- **We have been developing** a number of experimental methods for schizophrenia.
- **Over a number of years, we have been investigating** ways of reducing energy loss in this device.
- **We have been studying** ways of reducing energy loss.
- **We have been looking at** ways of reducing energy loss.

研究内容を説明する際は現在完了進行形（have been 〜ing）を用いる．これは，その研究が過去に始まり現在も進行中であることを示している．

> **Note** The easiest way of reminding the audience of your current research is with the phrase **We have been working on** + research topic. The pattern is **We have been working on** + (topic). This pattern refers to work that started some time ago and is ongoing. Another useful sentence is, **We have been looking at** + research topic.

3 Remind the audience of the presentation topic
発表テーマを再度述べる

It is common for presenters to **state the topic of the presentation again**. This is just **to remind the audience of the topic** and **to focus on what was studied**. Although this is just a short sentence, it is a very effective way of starting the summary.

発表テーマを改めて述べることで，聴衆が発表の内容を振り返りやすくなる．

Starting the summary: Steps 1-5　まとめを始める：ステップ 1〜5

本日は〜についてお話ししました．

- **Today, I talked about** water pollution in agricultural areas.
- **We looked at** water pollution in agricultural areas.
- **So, we looked at** water pollution in agricultural areas.
- **Today, I focused on** water pollution in agricultural areas.

> Probably, the easiest way of reminding the audience of the presentation topic is with the patterns **We looked at** + topic and **So, we looked at** + topic.

発表テーマを述べる際は，(So,) we looked at + topic とするのが最も簡単である．

4　Restate the objectives
研究目的を再度述べる

Briefly restating the objectives of the study will help the audience.

この研究は〜を明らかにすることを目的に行いました．

- **Our main objective (in this study) was to** measure nitrates in rivers.
- **The main aim (of this research) was to investigate** nitrates in rivers.
- **We wanted to analyze** the levels of nitrates in rivers.

研究目的を振り返る際は，3番目の例文のように wanted を用いるのが最も簡単である．複数の目的について言及する場合は，wanted を繰り返し使用しても問題ない．

> A quick and easy way of restating objectives is with the verb **wanted**.

- **We wanted to** analyse levels of nitrates, and **we also wanted to** test methods of reducing nitrates.

You can use the word **wanted** several times to introduce a number of objectives.

Part 5 ● Finishing your presentation　発表の終わり方

5 Restate research questions
疑問・仮説を再度述べる

It will help the audience if your **conclusion slide refers back to the research questions** that were posed at the beginning of the presentation.

この研究によってどのような疑問（リサーチクエスチョン）に答えようとしたのか，どのような仮説を検証しようとしたのかを改めて述べる．必要に応じて，疑問・仮説をスライドに記載するとよい．

（スライドを示しながら）この研究では，このような疑問に答えようとしました．

- **This is just to remind you of our research questions. What are the sources of nitrates in rivers** and **how can they be reduced?**
  (In this example and the ones that follow, research questions can be shown on the slide if necessary)
- **This was our research question.**
- **These were our research questions.**
- **I'd just like to remind you of our research questions, which were as follows.**
- **This was our research hypothesis.**
- **This was our hypothesis.**
- **So, our research hypothesis was that** sunlight is a reliable method of degrading polymers.

Example of functions 1-5

This is a combined example of functions 1-5. It shows how to start the summary of your presentation with just a few sentences.

Script(1〜5をつなげた原稿の例)

This is my last slide. We have been working on ways of improving water quality, and looked at water pollution in agricultural areas. We wanted to analyse the level of nitrates. Our research question was: How can nitrates be controlled effectively?

2 Introduce the findings, implications, and future work: Steps 6-11
研究結果のポイントや聴衆へのメッセージを述べる：ステップ 6〜11

6 Introduce the findings
結果を紹介する

Script(結果のまとめの例)

① Here are the results from the 15 institutions caring for the elderly that implemented the study program. ② We found that the average number of falls per patient decreased by more than 20 percent. ③ We also found that there was an improvement in patient mobility, balance, and general fitness. ④ Additionally, we found an increase in patients' wellbeing and general happiness.

Key sentences

6.1 Signal the start of the findings
結果の紹介を始めることを示す

The presenter begins by signaling the start of the findings.

こちらが本研究の主な結果です.

■ Here are the results from the 15 institutions caring for the elderly that implemented the study program.

  Examples
■ These are the findings / main results / main points from the program.
■ These are our main findings.

はじめに結果の紹介に入る合図として左記のように言う.

194　Part 5 ● Finishing your presentation　発表の終わり方

6.2 Stating the findings　結果を紹介する

～であることが明らかになりました.

■ **We found that** the average number of falls per patient decreased by more than 20 percent.

結果の要点を We found that などの能動態の文で紹介する.

> **Examples**

■ **Results showed that** there was a 20 percent reduction in falls.
■ **So, what we saw was** a 20 percent reduction in falls.
■ **So, we saw** a 20 percent reduction in falls.
■ **There was** a 20 percent reduction in falls.

6.3 Introducing more findings
結果をさらに紹介する（1）

また，～ということも分かりました.

■ **We also found that** there was an improvement in patient mobility, balance, and general fitness.

複数の結果を紹介する場合は, also, additionally, the other thing (that) we found was that などの表現を用いる.

> **Examples**

■ **The other thing (that) we found was that** patient mobility, balance, and general fitness improved.

6.4 Introducing additional findings
結果をさらに紹介する（2）

さらに，～についても明らかになりました.

■ **Additionally, we found** an increase in patients' wellbeing and general happiness.

> **Examples**

■ **Additionally, we found that** there was an increase in patients' wellbeing and general happiness.
■ **Another thing we found was** an increase in patients' wellbeing and general happiness.

2 Introduce the findings, implications, and future work: Steps 6-11
研究結果のポイントや聴衆へのメッセージを述べる：ステップ 6〜11

195

Note Presenters frequently use the following sentences to introduce their findings. <u>It was suggested that</u>, <u>It was concluded that</u>, <u>It was thought that</u>. These expressions are <u>too formal for oral presentations</u> and are used in written academic English only. It is better to introduce the findings with an active sentence starting with **we**. For example, <u>We found that</u>, <u>We also found that</u>.

結果の紹介の際に It was suggested that などの受動態の文を用いるのは，論文的で堅苦しい表現である．口頭発表では，We found that，We also found that など，we で始まる能動態の文にするとよい．

7 Explain the findings
結果から得られる結論を説明する

It is common for presenters to make **a general statement about their research findings**. This is a kind of overview that **puts the results in perspective** and gives the audience a more **global picture of the significance of the research/ study**.

主な結果を紹介した後は，その結果が何を示しているのか，その結果からどのような一般的な結論が導き出せるのかなどの考察を説明する．

7.1 Introduce the start of the explanation
説明を始めることを示す

Here the presenter signals the start of a general statement about the meaning of the results.

これらの結果は何を意味しているのでしょうか？

▌ <u>So, what do these results mean</u>?

> **Examples**

▌ <u>What is the significance of</u> these findings?

▌ <u>What is the meaning of</u> these results?

▌ <u>I'll summarize</u> the significance of these results.

はじめに説明に入る合図として左記のように言う．疑問形を用いることで聴衆の興味を引きつけることができる．

196　**Part 5** ● Finishing your presentation　発表の終わり方

7.2 Main message　結論を説明する

At this point, the presenter makes a comment on the findings presented so far in the form of a main message. Here are some useful expressions.

これらの結果は，〜であることを示しています．

■ **Taken together, these results tell us that** action taken at grass-roots level by local staff makes a significant difference in terms of a reduction in the number of falls, and also an increase in general health and wellbeing.

「これらの結果をまとめると」と言いたいときは taken together, taken as a whole, overall, all in all などの表現を用いる.「これらの結果は〜を示しています」は these results tell us that や these findings suggest that などとする.

Examples

■ **Taken together, these findings suggest that** action taken at grass-roots level by staff has more significant effects on patient wellbeing than top-down directives.

■ **Taken as a whole, this material shows** that action taken at grass-roots level by staff has more significant effects on patient wellbeing than top-down directives.

■ **Overall, these data indicate that** action taken at grass-roots level by staff has more significant effects on patient wellbeing than top-down directives.

■ **All in all, these findings indicate that** action taken at grass-roots level by staff on the ground has more significant effects on patient wellbeing than top-down directives.

Note A good way of emphasizing the main message is with the expressions, **Taken together, Taken as a whole, overall, all in all**. Please note that the verb in these sentences is in the present tense: **tell, suggest, show, indicate**. However, when you introduce the results the verb will be in the past tense. For example, **We found / We observed**. The verbs are in the past tense.

結果が何を示しているかを表す際に用いる動詞には tell, suggest, show, indicate などがある. 結果を紹介する場合は過去形（〜が分かった）であるが，結果から得られる結論を説明する場合は現在形（〜を示している）となることに注意する.

2 Introduce the findings, implications, and future work: Steps 6-11
研究結果のポイントや聴衆へのメッセージを述べる：ステップ 6〜11

8 State the take-home message
テイクホームメッセージを述べる

The take-home message is the main finding expressed as clearly as possible. It is the message that the presenter wants the audience to remember.

テイクホームメッセージ（take-home message）とは，聴衆に家に持ち帰ってほしいメッセージのことであり，その発表において最も伝えたいことをさす.

本日の発表のテイクホームメッセージは，～です.

▮ **This is the take-home message**. Local initiatives involving staff are more effective than top-down directives.

Examples

▮ **So, the take-home message is that** the numbers of falls can be significantly reduced by involving staff in the decision-making process.

▮ **Here is the take-home message**. Local initiatives involving staff are more effective than top-down directives.

▮ **Here is the take-away message.** The number of falls can be significantly reduced by involving staff on the ground in the decision-making process.

Note The expression **take-home message** means **take-away message**. Although the pattern is different, there is no difference in meaning. The expression **take-home message is more frequently used than take-away message.**

Take-home message は take-away（お持ち帰り）message ともよばれるが，take-home message のほうが一般的である.

198　Part 5 ● Finishing your presentation　発表の終わり方

9 Mention the implications
研究の意義を述べる

The word implications refers to the impact of the findings on the field. Here is an example.

> 最後にこの研究の結果が，その学問分野において，あるいは応用的・臨床的にどのような意義をもつのかを説明する．

Script（研究の意義を述べる例）

① What are the implications of these results? ② The main one is the obvious importance of local initiatives.

この研究の結果はどのような意義をもつでしょうか？

▮ **What are the implications of these results?**

Examples

▮ **What are the cost / nursing implications?**

▮ **What are the implications of this study for** healthcare of elderly people in institutions?

特に重要な点は，〜ということです．

▮ **The main one is the obvious importance of local initiatives.**

Examples

▮ **Local initiatives at the grass root level are more effective,** cost less and help to keep staff motivated.

▮ **The main implication is that** bottom-up initiatives involving front line staff are more effective in terms of cost and patient wellbeing than top-down directives.

▮ **I think it is clear that** initiatives at grass root level are more effective in terms of cost and patient wellbeing than top-down directives.

---

2 Introduce the findings, implications, and future work: Steps 6-11
研究結果のポイントや聴衆へのメッセージを述べる：ステップ 6〜11

10 Finishing with the expressions: I hope that, That's what I wanted to tell you about + topic, That's what I wanted to say about + topic　まとめを終える

In some cases, presenters use the following sentences to finish their presentations.

● I hope that this information has been of interest

本日の発表に興味をもっていただけたなら幸いです.

- I hope that you have found this data interesting.
- I hope that this presentation will promote interest in this largely under-researched field.
- I hope that this presentation will encourage others to look at ways of creating a safe environment in care homes.

● That is what I wanted to tell you today about (topic)

本日お話ししたかったことはこれで以上です.

- That is what I wanted to tell you today. I hope you found this data interesting.
- That is what I wanted to tell you about creating a safe environment in care homes.

● That is what I wanted to say about (topic)

本日お話ししたかったことはこれで以上です.

- That's what I wanted to say about (topic). I hope that you found this talk interesting.
- That is what I wanted to say about creating a safe environment in care homes.
- That is what I wanted to say about patient care. I think this aspect of care for the elderly deserves more attention.

> この後に今後の研究課題への言及や謝辞などは残っているが，発表の本論のまとめはこれで終わりとなる．まとめを終えることを示す表現として左記のように言う.

> I hope that は，「発表に興味をもっていただけたなら幸いです」「この発表が〜に興味をもつきっかけになれば幸いです」のような形で締めくくるのに用いる.

> That is what I wanted to tell you today about と That is what I wanted to say about はともに，発表内容が以上で終わりであることを示している.

200　Part 5 ● Finishing your presentation　発表の終わり方

- **That is what I wanted to say about** patient care. **I think** this aspect of care **merits more attention**.
- **That is what I wanted to say about** patient care. **I think** this aspect of care **necessitates further research/study**.
- **That is what I wanted to say today**. **I hope you found this data interesting**.
- **Those were/are the points I wanted to make today**.

11 Future work / Future directions
今後の研究課題を述べる

Most presenters include a statement about future work. The following sentences signal that you will talk about future work.

一通り発表内容のまとめを述べた後，今後の研究課題についても簡単に紹介する．

今後の研究課題についても簡単にご説明します．私達は今後～を行う予定です．

- **I'd (just) like to mention (our) future work**. **We plan to do** further experiments with lasers.
- **I'll (just) say a few words about future directions**. **We plan to do** further experiments with lasers.
- **As for future work, we plan to do** further experiments using lasers.
- **In terms of future work, we plan to do** further experiments using lasers.
- **Concerning future work, we plan to do** further experiments using lasers.

> **Note** In the above examples, the following 3 expressions are used to introduce future work: **As for future work**, **In terms of future work**, **Concerning future work**,

今後の研究課題の紹介を始める際は，As for future work, In terms of future work, Concerning future work などの表現が有用である．

2 Introduce the findings, implications, and future work: Steps 6-11
研究結果のポイントや聴衆へのメッセージを述べる：ステップ 6～11

201

Here I show how to give examples of future work using the following verbs: <u>plan</u>, <u>want</u>, <u>is</u>.

● Plan

次は〜を行う予定です．

- <u>We plan to do further experiments</u> using lasers.
- <u>We plan to do another study with</u> more subjects <u>focusing on</u> a wider range of OTC whitening products.
- <u>We are planning to investigate</u> the use of laser technology.
- <u>We are planning to do another study on</u> the incidence of relapse in people using OTC whitening products.
- <u>(As for future work), we are planning to do more experiments on</u> how to refine the system with a laser.
- <u>(Concerning future work), we are planning to do more experiments on</u> how to refine the system with a laser.
- <u>(In terms of future work), we plan to conduct further research on</u> OTC whitening products.

Plan（動詞）を用いて，**We plan to do** や **We are planning to do** のような形で，今後の研究計画を述べる．

 A common pattern is <u>We plan to do more work / more experiments / another study on</u> topic.

● Want

今後は〜について調べたいと思っております．

- <u>We want to</u> take further samples at lower temperatures.
- <u>We want to look at</u> ways of reducing interference.
- <u>We want to look at</u> ways of overcoming the above problems associated with institutionalized adults.

Want を用いる場合は，**We want to** の形で，今後行いたいと考えている研究の内容を紹介する．

● Is (to)

次の課題は〜です.

- ▌ <u>The next step is to</u> refine the system with laser technology.
- ▌ <u>The next stage (in this research) is to</u> refine the system with laser technology.
- ▌ <u>Our next goal is to</u> achieve higher yields in terms of production.
- ▌ <u>What we want to do next is to</u> develop a more robust system that can be used in colder environments.

Is を用いる場合は, is to (＋動詞) の形で,「次の課題は〜することです」のように言う.

> **Note** The expression **is to + verb** is usually preceded by the following expressions:
>
> - ▌ The next step
> - ▌ The next stage
> - ▌ Our next goal
> - ▌ The next part of this research
> - ▌ What we want to do next
> - ▌ What we plan to do next
>
> + is to + develop an improved system.

Please note the **usage of singular and plural** in the following expressions.

「今後の課題」や「今後の研究計画」と言うとき, work, research は単数形で, plans, projects, experiments, directions, perspectives は複数形で用いることに注意する.

1. <u>Usually singular</u>: Future work, future research

The words **work** and **research** are not used in the plural.

2. <u>Usually plural</u>: Future plans, future projects, future experiments, future directions, future perspectives

The words **plans**, **projects**, **experiments**, **directions** and **perspectives** are generally plural when talking about future work.

3 Finishing the presentation: Steps 12-16
発表を終える：ステップ 12〜16

12 Funding
研究助成に言及する

Recently, it is common for presenters to include information on funding.

最近は，発表の終わりに研究助成について言及するのが一般的である．

> この研究は○○基金の研究助成を受けて行いました．
>
> - **This research/study/work was supported by a grant from** the Ministry of Construction.
> - **I'd just like to mention that this research was supported by a grant from** the Sato Foundation.
> - **For this research, we obtained funding from** the Ministry of Education.
> - **For this research, we got funding from** the Ministry of Education.

研究助成について紹介する際は **be supported by a grant from** や **we obtained/got funding from** のように言う．Obtained のほうが got よりも改まった表現である．

 The word <u>obtained</u> is more formal than <u>got</u>. <u>Got</u> is widely used as it is informal and easy to say.

> （スライドにリストを表示しながら）この研究はこれらの研究助成を受けて行いました．
>
> - **You can see our funding sources here**. (Show a list of funding sources. It is not necessary to read them).
> - **Here are the sources of funding for this work**. (Show a list of funding sources. It is not necessary to read them).

利用した研究助成が複数ある場合は，スライドに研究助成のリストを提示したうえで左記のように述べてもよい．この場合，リストを1つ1つ読み上げる必要はない．

 Funding is always singular. You cannot say *fundings*.

Funding は常に単数形で使用し，*fundings* とはしないことに注意する．

13 Acknowledgments
謝辞を述べる

Here are some examples of how to introduce acknowledgments.

この研究にご協力いただいた皆様に感謝いたします.

▌ **I wish to thank the following people.** (+ a list of names and a photo)

続いて研究協力者や共同研究者への謝辞を述べる. その際の動詞はthank または acknowledge を用いる.

● Thank

▌ **I want to thank my coworkers at** the Institute of Health Science.

▌ **I'd like to thank my colleagues at** the Institute of Health Science.

▌ **I'd like to say a big thank you to** my coworkers at AIST.

口頭で謝辞を述べるのに合わせ, スライドに研究協力者のリストと写真を表示するとよい.

● Acknowledge

▌ **I'd like to acknowledge the following people.** (Show a list of people's names)

14 Signal the end of the presentation
結びの挨拶を述べる

It is important to signal the end of the presentation clearly. The shortest way of doing this is to say, **Thank you**. This is short for **Thank you for your attention**. Another option is, **That's all I have to say**. Some presenters shorten this to *That's all*, but this is too abrupt and rather informal.

Here are some examples.

結びの挨拶として聴衆へのお礼を述べる. Thank you for your attention と言うか, より簡単に Thank you でもよい.

Thank you の前に「本日の発表は以上です」(That's all I have to say) と言う場合もある.

3 Finishing the presentation: Steps 12-16　発表を終える：ステップ 12〜16

本日の発表は以上です．ご清聴ありがとうございました．

- Thank you.
- Thank you very much.
- Thank you for your attention.
- Thank you very much for your attention.
- That's all I have to say. Thank you for your attention.
- That covers what I wanted to say today. Thank you for your attention.
- That covers what I wanted to say about （topic）. Thank you for your attention.
- That concludes my presentation. Thank you for your attention.

Common errors──よくある間違い

× *Thanks*.
○ Thank you.
○ Thank you very much.

The word <u>thanks</u> is too informal and not suitable for an oral presentation at a conference.

Thanks はくだけた表現なので学会発表では避ける．

× *That's it*.
○ That is all I have to say.
○ That is all I have to say. Thank you for your attention.

The expression *That's it* is too informal for a conference presentation. If it is combined with another expression, it can be used, but it is still rather informal. For example, <u>That's it. Thank you very much for your attention</u>. Generally, I advise presenters to avoid the expression *That's it*.

That's it もくだけた表現であり，学会発表では避ける．他の表現と組み合わせて That's it. Thank you very much for your attention などとすれば使用可能ではあるが，それでもくだけた印象は残るため，基本的には使用しないほうがよい．

206　Part 5 ● Finishing your presentation　発表の終わり方

✗ *That's all.*
✗ *That's all for my presentation.*
○ Thank you.
○ Thank you for your attention.
○ That's all I have to say. Thank you for your time.
○ That's all I have to say. Thank you for your attention.
○ That concludes my presentation. Thank you.

That's all は必ず *I have to say* と組み合わせて *That's all I have to say* の形で用いる。*That's all* や *That's all for my presentation* はともに使用できない。

I am surprised that so many presenters use these expressions. *That's all.* / *That's all for my presentation*. Both are incorrect. If you use **That's all**, you must use the expression **I have to say**. For example, **That's all I have to say. Thank you for your attention**. Please avoid *That's all for my presentation*. It is incorrect and makes a bad impression.

✗ Thank you for **your** listening.
○ Thank you for listening.

「ご清聴ありがとうございました」を *Thank you for your listening* とするのは誤り。*Your* を削除して *Thank you for listening* とするか、*Thank you for your attention* とするのが正しい。*Attention* は単数形で用いることにも注意する。

In the above error, the problem is the expression *your listening*. It is possible to say, **Thank you for your attention**. But, *Thank you for your listening* is not correct.

✗ Thank you for your **attentions**.
○ Thank you for your **attention**.

The word attention is always singular and never plural.

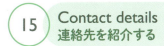

Contact details
連絡先を紹介する

In some cases, presenters mention their contact details and show their email addres on the screen.

3 Finishing the presentation: Steps 12-16　発表を終える：ステップ 12〜16

（スライドにメールアドレスを表示して）こちらが私の連絡先です. 興味のある方はどうそお気兼ねなくご連絡ください.

- ∎ **Here are my contact details. Please feel free to get in contact.**
- ∎ **Here are my contact details. If you are interested in this study or would like to have any more information, please get in contact.**

連絡先を紹介する際は，スライドにメールアドレスを表示したうえで左記のように言う.

16 Invite questions
質問を呼びかける

Most sessions have a chairperson who will handle the question and answer session. In these cases, it is unnecessary to invite questions. In cases where there is no chairperson, you can invite questions in the following way.

何か質問はございますか?

- ∎ **I'd be happy to take any questions you might have.**
- ∎ **I'd be happy to answer any questions.**
- ∎ **I'll take questions now.**
- ∎ **Are there any questions or comments?**
- ∎ **Does anyone have any questions or comments?**

質問を呼びかけるのは通常座長の役割であるが，座長がいない場合には発表者自らが左記のような表現で質問を呼びかける.

Note A lot of presenters and people who act as a chairperson use the following pattern. *Any question?* This is incorrect because the word **question** should be plural. **Any questions?** But this not a full sentence and sounds very casual. The full sentence is as follows: **Are there any questions?** Sometimes this is extended to, **Are there any questions or comments? / Does anyone have any questions or comments?**

質問を呼びかける際, *Any question?* とするのは誤り. Question を複数形にして **Any questions?** とするのが正しい. ただし, これもややくだけた表現であるため, **Are there any questions?** としたほうが丁寧である.

質問だけではなく, コメントも加えて **questions or comments** とする場合もある.

208　Part 5 ● Finishing your presentation　発表の終わり方

Part 6

How to create a clear summary slide and an audience-friendly script

分かりやすいまとめスライドの作り方，説明の仕方

In this part, I show how to change an existing summary slide with several serious problems to an easy to understand slide with a script that supports the main points in the slide. You will see that the summary is changed from something that is too wordy and difficult to understand to something that is more accessible.

In this section, I cover 2 summary slides, each of which consists of 5 parts.

1. **The slide before revision**
2. **How to make your slide more accessible by using less formal English**
3. **The revised slide**
4. **The script for introducing the information on the summary slide**
5. **Summary script: Functions and more examples**

　発表の最後には，「まとめスライド」を提示し，発表内容の要点を振り返ります．この際，ただ文章を羅列しただけのスライドでは，聴衆にとって分かりやすいまとめとはいえません．この章では，2つの例を通じて，簡潔で見やすいまとめスライドを作成する方法を示します．また，まとめスライドを説明する際の原稿作成のポイントについても併せて解説します．

Summary slide example 1
まとめスライドの改善例（1）

First, let's look at the summary slide in its original form. Please spend a minute or two reading through the material on the slide. Try to identify the main points that the presenter wants to make.

1.1 The slide before revision
改善前のまとめスライド

Summary

The authors found snacking significantly increases the child's risk of developing dental caries, in some cases in excess of 20 percent. The crucial factors in elevated risk of caries were established as frequency, that is to say, the number of times foods with high levels of sugar were consumed, and consistency of items consumed, that is thickness and smoothness. Moreover, risk of cavities depended to a greater degree on consistency than amount consumed. The role of sealants in preventing caries in early childhood will be the subject of a future study.

This summary slide has the following issues.

▌ There are too many words.
▌ There is too much information.
▌ There is no space between sentences.
▌ The main points are not clear.
▌ The English is too formal for an oral presentation.
▌ The audience will not have time to read or understand the information.

Part 6 ● How to create a clear summary slide and an audience-friendly script
分かりやすいまとめスライドの作り方，説明の仕方

1.2 How to make your summary slide more accessible by using less formal English
格式張らない英語を使って，読みやすいスライドに直す方法

One of the problems with this slide is that the **English is too formal**. Here I show how to **reduce the formality of the English and create a slide that is simple and easy to follow**. In the examples below, the original sentence is shown. Next, **formal expressions are shown on the left** and **less formal expressions on the right**. After that, **the revised sentence is shown in full**.

前ページのまとめスライドは，文章量・情報量が多すぎるため，聴衆は全体を読み切ることができず，どこが要点なのかがつかめない．また，使われている英語も，論文調の格式張った表現であり，学会発表に適したものではない．

The authors found snacking significantly increases the child's risk of developing dental caries, in some cases in excess of 20 percent.

Formal expressions	Less formal expressions
▌ The authors found	▌ We found that
▌ significantly increases	▌ increases a lot
▌ the child's risk of developing dental caries	▌ the child's risk of getting tooth decay
▌ in excess of 20 percent.	▌ by more than 20 percent

We found that snacking increases the child's risk of getting tooth decay a lot, in some cases by more than 20 percent.

❶ Summary slide example 1 まとめスライドの改善例（1）

The crucial factors in elevated risk of caries were established as frequency, that is to say, the number of times foods with high levels of sugar were consumed, and consistency of items consumed, that is thickness and smoothness.

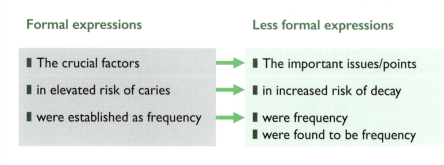

Formal expressions	Less formal expressions
▍ The crucial factors	▍ The important issues/points
▍ in elevated risk of caries	▍ in increased risk of decay
▍ were established as frequency	▍ were frequency ▍ were found to be frequency

Note The expression **established as** has been deleted. The revised phrases are as follows: **were frequency** / **were found to be frequency**

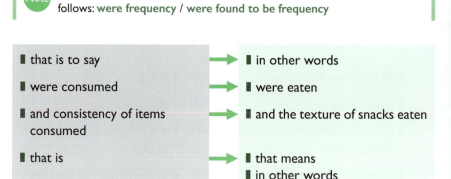

▍ that is to say	▍ in other words
▍ were consumed	▍ were eaten
▍ and consistency of items consumed	▍ and the texture of snacks eaten
▍ that is	▍ that means ▍ in other words

The important issues in increased risk of decay were frequency, in other words, the number of times snacks with high levels of sugar were eaten and the texture of the snack eaten, that means thickness and consistency.

Moreover, risk of cavities depended to a greater degree on consistency than amount consumed.

Formal expressions	Less formal expressions
▌ Moreover	▌ Also ▌ In addition
▌ cavities	▌ decay
▌ to a greater degree on	▌ more on
▌ consumed	▌ eaten

Also risk of decay depended more on consistency / texture than the amount eaten.

The role of sealants in preventing caries in early childhood will be the subject of a future study.

Formal expressions	Less formal expressions
▌ will be the subject of a future study	▌ As for future work, we plan to do a study on

As for future work, we plan to do a study on sealants as a way of preventing tooth decay in children.

▌ Summary slide example I　まとめスライドの改善例（1）

1.3 The revised slide
改善後のまとめスライド

Below you will see the revised slide, which now consists of notes on all the main points.

> ## Summary
>
> - Snacking **increases the risk of caries** in children
> - Sometimes **in excess of 20 percent**
> - Factors affecting risk: **1. frequency 2. consistency**
> - **Risk depends more on consistency than amount eaten**
> - **Future work: Using sealants as a way of preventing tooth decay** in children

1.4 Script for explaining the information on the summary slide
まとめスライド説明用の原稿

This is the script for the summary slide. It is shown as a single paragraph.

Script(上記まとめスライド説明用の原稿の例)

① I would like to finish with a brief summary. ② We looked at the effect of snacking on risk of children getting tooth decay. ③ We found that snacking increases the child's risk of getting tooth decay. In some cases, this can be more than 20 percent. ④ We also found that there are two main factors that seem to affect risk. One is frequency. This means, the number of times the child snacks. ⑤ The other is consistency of the snack. Consistency, as I have already mentioned, is related to how much of the snack gets stuck between the teeth and attached to the surface of the teeth. ⑥ Finally, I'd like to stress that our results show that consistency is a greater risk than the amount of snacks eaten. ⑦ As for future work, we plan to do a study on sealants as a way of preventing tooth decay in children. ⑩ That's all I have to say. Thank you for your attention.

Summary script: functions and more examples
まとめスライド説明用原稿の例文

Here the main functions used to explain the summary slide are listed with further examples.

以下，前ページの説明用原稿中の各文について，似たような意味をもつ例文を紹介する．まとめを述べる際に用いられる表現のさらに詳しい解説と例文については，Part. 5 を参照．

1. Signal the start of the summary　まとめに入ることを示す

最後に，本日の発表のまとめをいたします．

- <u>I would like to finish with</u> a brief summary.

まとめに入る合図として，左記のように言う．

Examples
- This is my last slide.
- This is a summary.

2. Remind the audience of the study aims
研究の目的を振り返る

この研究の目的は，～することでした．

- <u>We looked at</u> the effect of snacking on risk of children getting tooth clecay.

最初に研究の目的を改めて述べることで，聴衆が発表の全体像を振り返りやすくなる．

Examples
- <u>We studied</u> the effect of snacking on risk of children getting tooth clecay.
- <u>We focused on</u> the effect of snacking on risk of children getting tooth clecay.
- <u>We investigated</u> the effect of snacking on risk of children getting tooth clecay.

3. Introduce the main findings　主な結果を紹介する．

～であることが分かりました．

- <u>We found that</u> snacking increases the child's risk of getting tooth decay. In some cases, this can be more than 20 percent.

続いて，この研究によって明らかになった主な結果を述べる．

1　Summary slide example 1　まとめスライドの改善例 (1)

Examples

▌ **This data shows that** snacking increases the child's risk of getting tooth decay. In some cases, this can be more than 20 percent.

▌ **So, the data shown here tells us that** snacking increases the risk of tooth decay in children. In some cases, this can be more than 20 percent.

▌ **So, the information shown here means that** snacking increases the risk of tooth decay in children. In some cases, this can be more than 20 percent.

▌ **So, the data shown here indicates that** snacking increases the risk of caries in children. In some cases, this can be more than 20 percent.

▌ **From this study, we concluded that** snacking increases the risk of caries in children. In some cases, this can be more than 20 percent.

4. Introduce more detailed findings（1）
結果をさらに詳しく紹介する（1）

また，〜ということも明らかになりました．

▌ **We also found that** there are two main factors that seem to affect risk.

> さらに他の内容についても言及する場合は，**We also found** や **In addition,** を用いる.

Examples

▌ **In addition, we found that** there are two main factors that seem to affect risk.

▌ **Additionally, we found that** there are two main factors that seem to affect risk.

▌ **Another thing that we found was that** there are two main factors that seem to affect risk.

216　Part 6 ● How to create a clear summary slide and an audience-friendly script
分かりやすいまとめスライドの作り方，説明の仕方

これは言い換えれば，〜ということです．

- One is frequency. **This means,** the number of times the child snacks.

  Examples

- **In other words,** the number of times the child snacks.
- **Frequency refers to** the number of times the child snacks.

専門用語などを他の言葉に言い換えて説明する際は，左記のように言う．

5. Introduce more detailed findings（2）
結果をさらに詳しく紹介する（2）

1. Adding another point

他の要因としては，〜があります．

- **The other（factor）is** consistency of the snack.

  Examples

- **The other issue is** consistency of the snack.
- **The other key factor is** consistency of the snack.

2. Reminding the audience of information already presented

先ほど申し上げたとおり，〜．

- Consistency, **as I have already mentioned,** is related to how much of the snack gets stuck between the teeth and attached to the surface of the teeth.

  Examples

- **As I said,** consistency of the snack is related to how much of the snack gets stuck between the teeth and attached to the surface of the teeth.
- **As I told you** consistency of the snack is related to how much of the snack gets stuck between the teeth and attached to the surface of the teeth.
- **As I pointed out,** consistency of the snack is related to how much of the snack gets stuck between the teeth and attached to the surface of the teeth.

既に一度説明したことに再度言及する際は，As I have already mentioned, や As I said, に続けて言うとよい．

Summary slide example 1　まとめスライドの改善例（1）

6. Introduce the main message　聴衆に一番伝えたいことを述べる

特に重要なポイントは，〜ということです．

- **<u>Finally, I'd like to stress that</u>** our results show that consistency is a greater risk than the amount of snacks eaten.

> **Examples**

- **<u>Our main finding was that</u>** consistency is a greater risk than the amount of snacks eaten.
- **<u>The most important finding was that</u>** consistency is a greater risk than the amount of snacks eaten.
- **<u>The key finding was that</u>** consistency is a greater risk than the amount of snacks eaten.
- **<u>The take-home message is that</u>** consistency is a greater risk than the amount of snacks eaten.

聴衆に最も強調して伝えたいことを述べる．このようなメッセージは，テイクホームメッセージ（**take-home message**）ともよばれる．

7. Introduce future work　今後の研究課題を述べる

今後は〜についての研究を進めていくつもりです．

- **<u>As for future work, we plan to do a study on</u>** sealants as a way of preventing tooth decay in children.

> **Examples**

- **<u>I'd just like to mention (our) future research plans. We plan to carry out further tests on</u>** the effects of sealing teeth in young children.
- **<u>I'd just like to mention that we are now conducting a further study on</u>** prevention of tooth decay in children using sealants.
- **<u>The aim of our future work is to conduct further tests on</u>** the effects of sealing teeth in young children.
- **<u>As for future work, we plan to do a study on</u>** sealants as a way of preventing tooth decay in children.
- **<u>The next step in this research is to carry out further tests on</u>** the effects of sealing teeth in young children.

まとめの最後は，今回の研究の結果を受け，今後どのような研究を行っていくつもりかを紹介する．

8. Acknowledgments 謝辞

 Functions 8~10 are not included in the summary slide, but I have listed them here because they are useful examples.

8~10 はまとめスライドに含める内容ではないが，まとめ同様に発表の最後に読み上げる内容である．

この研究にご協力いただいた皆様に感謝いたします．

- **I want to thank the people who have been involved in this work.** (show a list of people's names and a photo)
  - Examples
- **I would like to thank my coworkers who have contributed to this work.**
- **I'd like to acknowledge** my coworkers who have contributed to this work.

共同研究者など，研究に関わった人達への感謝の言葉を述べる．その際，共同研究者の名前のリストや写真をスライドに表示するとよい．

9. Mention funding 研究助成への言及

この研究は○○基金の研究助成を受けて行いました．

- **This research was funded by** the Ministry of Health, Welfare and Labor.
  - Examples
- **For this project we are getting funding from** the Dutch Program for Tissue Engineering.
- **We gratefully acknowledge the financial support of** Lion Corporation.

研究助成を受けて行った研究の場合は，その名称などを紹介する．

10. Thank the audience 聴衆へのお礼

ご清聴ありがとうございました．

- **That's all I have to say**. **Thank you for your attention**.
  - Examples
- **That concludes my presentation**. **Thank you.**
- **That covers everything I wanted to say**. **Thank you for your attention**.

最後に聴衆へのお礼を述べ，発表を締めくくる．

Summary slide example 1　まとめスライドの改善例（1）

2 Summary slide example 2
まとめスライドの改善例（2）

Let's start by looking at the slide in its original form. Please read through the information on the slide and identify the main points.

2.1 The summary slide before revision
改善前のまとめスライド

Summary

Our objective was to improve the physical and mental health of at risk people in areas with high levels of social issues.

Low-cost interventions for cardio-vascular disease and diabetes were investigated. Exercise, diet, and general health were focused on. Online and face-to-face materials were developed, including questionnaires, apps, automated reminders and community spaces, all of which could be accessed and submitted online.

It was found that after 6 months the following improved: mood, energy levels, mental function, blood pressure and BMI.

It was concluded that low-cost interventions focusing on at risk patients are effective in reducing the risk of serious diseases such as heart disease and diabetes. It was also suggested that low-cost interventions could be used effectively in combination with standard treatments. Ways of increasing patient access to low-cost interventions are currently being studied.

2.2 How to make the summary slide more accessible by using less formal English
格式張らない英語を使って，読みやすいスライドに直す方法

Our objective was to improve the physical and mental health of at risk people in areas with high levels of social issues.

Formal expressions

- Our objective was to improve

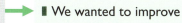

Informal expressions

- We wanted to improve
- Our aim was to improve

We wanted to improve the physical and mental health of at risk people in areas with high levels of social issues.

Low-cost interventions for cardio-vascular disease and diabetes were investigated.

Formal expressions

- were investigated

Informal expressions

- We looked at low-cost interventions
- We focused on low-cost interventions
- We investigated low-cost interventions
- We studied low-cost interventions

We looked at low-cost interventions for cardio-vascular disease and diabetes.

2 Summary slide example 2　まとめスライドの改善例 (2)

Exercise, diet, and general health were focused on.

Formal expressions

▌ were focused on

Informal expressions

▌ We looked at

▌ We focused on

We also looked at exercise, diet, and general health.

Online and face-to-face materials were developed, including questionnaires, apps, automated reminders and community spaces, all of which could be accessed and submitted online.

Formal expressions

▌ were developed

Informal expressions

▌ We made

▌ We created

We made online and face-to-face materials, including questionnaires, apps, automated reminders and community spaces, all of which could be accessed and submitted online.

It was found that after 6 months the following improved: mood, energy levels, mental function, blood pressure and BMI.

Formal expressions

▌ It was found that

Informal expressions

▌ We found that

▌ We concluded that

We found that after 6 months the following improved: mood, energy levels, mental function, blood pressure and BMI.

It was concluded that low-cost interventions focusing on at risk patients are effective in reducing the risk of serious diseases such as heart disease and diabetes.

Formal expressions

Informal expressions

▌ It was concluded

▌ We found that
▌ We concluded that

We found that low-cost interventions focusing on at risk patients are effective in reducing the risk of serious diseases such as heart disease and diabetes.

It was also suggested that low-cost interventions could be used effectively in combination with standard treatments.

Formal expressions

Informal expressions

▌ It was also suggested

▌ We also found

▌ Additionally, we found

Additionally, we found that low-cost interventions could be used effectively in combination with standard treatments.

Ways of increasing patient access to low-cost interventions are currently being studied.

Formal expressions

Informal expressions

▌ are currently being studied

▌ We are now working on ways of

We are now working on ways of increasing patient access to low-cost interventions.

2 Summary slide example 2　まとめスライドの改善例（2）

2.3 The revised slide
改善後のまとめスライド

Summary

Aims Improve the physical and mental health of at risk people in areas with high levels of social issues.

Approach Investigate the benefits of low-cost online approaches to interventions for diseases such as heart disease and diabetes, focusing on exercise, diet and general health.

Online interventions Questionnaires, apps, automated reminders, communal online support spaces.

Health benefits After 6 months, the following improved: mood, energy levels, mental functions, blood pressure and BMI.

Take-home message Low-cost online interventions are effective in reducing the risk of serious diseases such as heart disease and diabetes, and can be used effectively in combination with standard treatments.

Future directions How to increase patient access to low-cost interventions.

2.4 Script for introducing the summary slide
まとめスライド説明用の原稿

Here is the script for introducing the information on the above slide.

Script（前ページのまとめスライド説明用原稿の例）

① This is a summary. ② We wanted to improve the physical and mental health of at risk people in areas with high levels of social issues. ③ We looked at the benefits of low-cost online approaches and face-to-face interventions for CVD and diabetes, focusing on exercise, diet, and general health.

④ We used online interviews as well as questionnaires, apps, automated reminders and community spaces. ⑤ Here are the main results. We found that after 6 months, the following improved: mood, energy levels, blood pressure and BMI. ⑥ This is the main message. We found that low-cost interventions focusing on at risk individuals were effective in reducing the risk of heart disease, diabetes and other serious diseases. ⑦ Additionally, we found that low-cost interventions could be used effectively in combination with standard treatments. ⑧ I'd like to mention future directions. We are now working on ways of increasing patient access to low-cost interventions.

2.5 Summary script: functions and examples
まとめスライド説明用原稿の例文

1. Signal the start of the summary　まとめに入ることを示す

こちらが本日の発表のまとめです.

- **This is a summary**.

> **Examples**

- **This is my last slide**.
- **I'd like to go over** the main points.
- **These are the main points I covered today**.
- **I'm going to summarize** my presentation.

> まとめの各ステップで用いる表現については, まとめスライド改善例 (1) (pp. 214〜219) および Part. 5 も参照.

> まとめに入る合図として, まとめスライドを示しながら左記のように言う.

2. Restate the objectives　研究の目的を再度述べる

～を目的にこの研究を行いました.

- **<u>We wanted to</u>** improve the physical and mental health of at risk people in areas with high levels of social issues.

Examples

- **<u>The main aim was to</u>** find ways to improve the physical and mental health of at risk people in areas with high levels of social issues.
- **<u>We looked at</u>** ways of improving the physical and mental health of at risk people in areas with high levels of social issues.

はじめに研究の目的を振り返る.

3. Introduce the topic　テーマを紹介する

～について, 特に～を中心に調べました.

- **<u>We looked at</u>** the benefits of low-cost online approaches and face-to-face interventions for CVD and diabetes, **<u>focusing on</u>** exercise, diet, and general health.

Examples

- **<u>We analyzed</u>** the benefits of low-cost online approaches and face-to-face interventions for CVD and diabetes, **<u>focusing on</u>** exercise, diet, and general health.
- **<u>We investigated</u>** the benefits of low-cost online approaches and face-to-face interventions for CVD and diabetes, **<u>focusing on</u>** exercise, diet, and general health.
- **<u>We assessed</u>** the benefits of low-cost online approaches and face-to-face interventions for CVD and diabetes, **<u>focusing on</u>** exercise, diet, and general health.
- **<u>We considered</u>** the benefits of low-cost online approaches and face-to-face interventions for CVD and diabetes, **<u>focusing on</u>** exercise, diet, and general health.

発表のテーマを再度紹介する.

4. Introduce the methods　研究方法を紹介する

～という手法を用いました.

■ **We used** online interviews as well as questionnaires, apps, automated reminders and community spaces.

研究の方法を簡単に振り返る.

Examples

■ **We employed** online interviews as well as questionnaires, apps, automated reminders and community spaces.

■ **We made use of** online interviews as well as question-naires, apps, automated reminders and community spaces.

5. Introduce the results　結果を紹介する

こちらが主な結果です.

■ **Here are the main results**.（We found that）after 6 months, the following improved: mood, energy levels, blood pressure and BMI.

研究結果のうち，主なものを簡潔に紹介する.

Examples

■ **These are the main results**. After 6 months, the follow-ing improved: mood, energy levels, blood pressure and BMI.

■ **This is what we found**. We found that after 6 months, the following improved: mood, energy levels, blood pressure and BMI.

■ **These are the main findings**.（We found that）after 6 months, the following improved: mood, energy levels, blood pressure and BMI.

■ **I'll just run through the main results**.（We found that）after 6 months, the following improved: mood, energy levels, blood pressure and BMI.

■ **I'll just go over the main results**.（We found that）after 6 months, the following improved: mood, energy levels, blood pressure and BMI.

2　**Summary slide example 2**　まとめスライドの改善例（2）

6. Introduce the main message　聴衆へのメッセージを述べる

特に重要なのは，〜ということです．

- **This is the main message**.（We found that）low-cost interventions focusing on at risk individuals were effective in reducing the risk of heart disease, diabetes and other serious diseases.

  `Examples`

- **This is the take-home message**.（We found that）low-cost interventions focusing on at risk individuals were effective in reducing the risk of heart disease, diabetes and other serious diseases.

- **Taken together, these results show that** low-cost interventions focusing on at risk individuals are effective in reducing the risk of heart disease, diabetes and other serious diseases.

- **We concluded that** low-cost interventions focusing on at risk individuals are effective in reducing the risk of heart disease, diabetes and other serious diseases.

研究結果をもとに，聴衆に対して特に強調して伝えたいこと（take-home message）を述べる.

7. Add additional results　さらに結果を紹介する

さらに，〜ということも分かりました．

- **Additionally, we found** that low-cost interventions could be used effectively in combination with standard treatments.

  `Examples`

- **We also think that** such interventions can be used effectively in combination with standard treatments.

- **We also feel that** such interventions can be used effectively in combination with standard treatments.

- **These results also suggest / show that** such interventions can be used effectively in combination with standard treatments.

他の重要な結果についても紹介する.

228　**Part 6** ● How to create a clear summary slide and an audience-friendly script
分かりやすいまとめスライドの作り方，説明の仕方

8. Refer to future work　今後の研究に言及する

今後の研究についてもお話しします．現在，私達は〜に関する研究を進めています．

- **I'd like to mention future directions. We are now working on** ways of increasing patient access to low-cost interventions.

  Examples

- **I'd just like to mention future directions. We plan to carry out a study on** ways of increasing patient access to low-cost interventions.

- **I'll just say a few words about future directions. We plan to carry out a study on** ways of increasing patient access to low-cost interventions.

- **As for future directions, we plan to carry out a further study on** ways of increasing patient access to low-cost interventions.

- **In terms of future work, we plan to carry out a further study on** ways of increasing patient access to low-cost interventions.

- **The next step in this research is to carry out a study on** ways of increasing patient access to low-cost interventions.

最後に，今後の研究課題や現在進めている研究の概要についても言及する．

9. Finish the presentation　発表を終える

本日の発表は以上です．ご清聴ありがとうございました．

- **That's all I have to say. Thank you for your attention.**

  Examples

- **Thank you.**
- **Thank you for your time.**
- **Thank you very much for your attention.**

発表を締めくくるときは左記のように言う．

【著者略歴】
C.S.Langham

1976 年　ハダースフィールド大学卒業
1982 年　ケント大学大学院修了
2000 年　日本大学歯学部教授（英語）
2020 年　日本大学特任教授

国際学会 English　口頭発表
研究発表のための英語プレゼンテーション　ISBN978-4-263-43364-5

2019 年 12 月 20 日　第 1 版第 1 刷発行
2025 年 3 月 10 日　第 1 版第 3 刷発行

　　　　　著　者　C. S. Langham
　　　　　発行者　白　石　泰　夫
　　　　　発行所　医歯薬出版株式会社

〒113-8612　東京都文京区本駒込 1-7-10
TEL.　(03)5395-7638(編集)・7630(販売)
FAX.　(03)5395-7639(編集)・7633(販売)
https://www.ishiyaku.co.jp/
郵便振替番号 00190-5-13816

乱丁，落丁の際はお取り替えいたします　　印刷・あづま堂印刷／製本・愛千製本所
© Ishiyaku Publishers, Inc., 2019. Printed in Japan

本書の複製権・翻訳権・翻案権・上映権・譲渡権・貸与権・公衆送信権（送信可能化権を含む）・口述権は，医歯薬出版(株)が保有します．
本書を無断で複製する行為（コピー，スキャン，デジタルデータ化など）は，「私的使用のための複製」などの著作権法上の限られた例外を除き禁じられています．また私的使用に該当する場合であっても，請負業者等の第三者に依頼し上記の行為を行うことは違法となります．

JCOPY ＜出版者著作権管理機構 委託出版物＞
本書をコピーやスキャン等により複製される場合は，そのつど事前に出版者著作権管理機構（電話 03-5244-5088，FAX 03-5244-5089，e-mail：info@jcopy.or.jp）の許諾を得てください．

大好評発売中 ●「国際学会 English」シリーズ
英語の学会 もう怖くない！

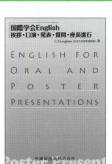

国際学会 English
挨拶・口演・発表・質問・座長進行

C.S.Langham 著

累計3万部突破のロングセラー．
学会会場に持って行きやすいハンディサイズ！

■ B6判／210頁／2色　■ 定価 2,750円(本体 2,500円＋税 10%)
ISBN978-4-263-43333-1

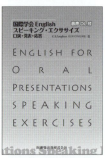

国際学会 English
スピーキング・エクササイズ
口演・発表・応答 音声 DL 付

C.S.Langham 著

音声DL付き！ 口頭発表で使うさまざまな表現を，
聞いて・話してマスターするための一冊！

■ A5判／120頁／2色　■ 定価 3,300円(本体 3,000円＋税 10%)
ISBN978-4-263-43368-3

国際学会 English
ポスター発表

C.S.Langham 著

ポスタープレビュー，発表，質疑応答まで，
ポスター発表のあらゆる場面で役立つ一冊！

■ A5判／128頁／2色　■ 定価 3,080円(本体 2,800円＋税 10%)
ISBN978-4-263-43354-6

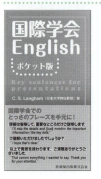

国際学会 English
ポケット版

C.S.Langham 著

ポスター大好評の「国際学会 English」シリーズから，特に便利な例文
を精選して1冊にまとめました．ポケットに入れておいて，いざという
ときに頼りになります！

■ A6判変／176頁／2色　■ 定価 2,420円(本体 2,200円＋税 10%)
ISBN978-4-263-43367-6

医歯薬出版株式会社

〒113-8612 東京都文京区本駒込1-7-10　TEL.03-5395-7630　FAX.03-5395-7633　https://www.ishiyaku.co.jp/